Healthy Mouth, Healthy Body

The Natural Dental Program for Total Wellness

Victor Zeines, D.D.S., M.S., FAGD

KENSINGTON BOOKS
http://www.kensingtonbooks.com

KENSINGTON BOOKS are published by

Kensington Publishing Corp.
850 Third Avenue
New York, NY 10022

ISBN 1-57566-589-1

First Kensington Printing: October, 2000
10 9 8 7 6 5 4 3 2 1

Printed in the United States of America

This book is dedicated to my father, professor Ben Zeines, who took all the first steps. To my mom, Bella, who was always there; my sons, Sam and David, who never knew what "junk foods" were and are the better for it, and to Kim, who endured hearing about this book for years.

ACKNOWLEDGMENTS

I would like to acknowledge one of my first teachers, Alec Rubin, who helped me start a holistic practice, and nutritional pioneers, Royal Lee, Weston Price, Melvin Pagen, Harold Hawkins, and many others. Thanks to my office staff, Donna, Linda, Karen, and Julie, for giving me such incredible support. Thanks to Lee Heiman and Claire Gerus, my editors and sometime teachers at Kensington Publishing, and to Les Sussman, who helped put it all together.

Contents

Introduction: From Milky Ways to Holistic Dentistry

As a kid growing up in a lower-middle-class family in the suburbs of New York City, I always hated going to the dentist.

I'll never forget one visit to my dentist where I actually prayed he wouldn't see the sweat dripping from my palms to the floor—that's how scared I was.

Years later, much to my surprise, I was actually on my way to *becoming* a dentist! My best friend decided to apply to dental school, and said, "Let's go together." Still undecided about a career, I applied to dental school. After graduation, I received an excellent internship at the Eastman Dental Clinic in Rochester, New York, considered the "Mayo Clinic" of dentistry.

This clinic accepted only two students each year from the United States—the rest of the interns were chosen from throughout the world—and I was one of the two domestic selections.

The internship didn't pay very well, so I began working at night at a nearby Medicaid clinic.

Here, I saw what an inadequate diet could do to a person's teeth. A few years later, I got a job with another Medicaid clinic—this one in the Bronx. One day the owner of the clinic introduced me to a dentist friend of his—Dr. Bruce Milner. He thought the two of us would get along well, and we did! Eventually, we opened our own dental clinic.

Although I enjoyed working with my patients, I felt that I really wasn't doing enough for them. I'd put in a filling, and a few months later, those same patients would come back with more decay. There was no medicine involved—no real healing. It was simple repair work.

Feeling discouraged, I quit dentistry and became a psychotherapist in New York City.

In therapy, I discovered much about myself as well as about other people. One important thing I discovered was that if you changed a person's diet, you could change his or her moods. A lot of my patients were scared and angry, but it wasn't a psychological problem—it was because they were hypoglycemic—suffering from low blood sugar.

I began to wonder whether a better diet could prevent dental problems, and I even went back to NYU to talk to some of my professors about it.

The response was discouraging, and I put my inquiries on the back burner. I decided to return to dentistry in 1975, and opened an office in Manhattan on Fifty-seventh Street.

One day I asked myself, "What will happen if I start giving my patients some vitamins?" There were a number of excellent vitamin manufacturers that were happy to talk to me about nutrition. So I hooked up with one and became very well versed on the subject.

Now a new door had opened up for me. I realized that there was a whole world of alternative healing out there that I didn't know anything about. I started taking courses in acupuncture.

I then studied acupressure and kinesiology, and that taught me many things about the human body. Through my new studies, I became aware that each part of the body is part of an integrated self, a complete piece of equipment that must function in perfect harmony.

One day I walked into a health food store and was astonished to find two books written by dentists on nutrition and other holistic modalities—*Diet and Disease* by E. Cheraskin, and *Nutrition and Physical Degeneration* by Weston Price.

These books had been written in the late 1930s and early 1940s and they described the exact kind of healing I wanted to do. Yet none of these holistic techniques had ever been mentioned in dental school on any level.

Now I began taking chiropractic courses, because these healers were willing to incorporate diet and nutrition into their treatment. I read about detoxology and nutrition, and came to understand how stress could affect a person's immune system and physical well-being.

I also began to learn how to treat my patients better—as people, not impersonally as I was trained to do in dental school.

I realized that all this knowledge could be applied to dentistry, and decided that to be the best I could in my field, I would have to aim high—to travel a different road than mainstream dentists. I had to see myself as a healer—not a tooth repairman.

In 1978, I met an incredible man named Gary Null. Gary is a medical researcher, author, and radio talk show host. He was—and still is—critical of conventional medicine, and at the time I met him he was speaking out about the benefits of natural methods of healing.

I began appearing on his radio talk shows, where we began to hear negative things about fillings containing mercury. Then a dentist named Dr. Hal Huggins spoke out about the potential toxicity of these fillings.

Gary and I began gathering more and more information about mercury from patients across the country.

In 1980, I began to observe that if I took the mercury fillings out of my patients' teeth, their health would improve. I'd hear such reports as, "My allergies are getting better," "I'm getting fewer colds," and similar stories.

I began to use vitamins, minerals, and herbal combinations to clean out my patients' systems after I had removed the mercury from their teeth. I also used herbs such as goldenseal, cayenne, garlic, and myrrh for patients who needed periodontal, or gum, surgery. Although those concoctions tasted odd and turned their teeth a little yellow, they healed the gums and—best of all—made surgery unnecessary.

By then I was a Fellow of the Academy of General Dentistry, and had decided to take more courses in periodontal therapy. I remember going to one class and raising my hand. I stood up and said, "I've been treating my patients the past two years with herbs." There was dead silence in the room. Then the lecturer looked at me and said, "Well, that's nice, Victor," and immediately changed the subject.

I felt better when, after the course, two or three dentists came over to me and said, "We'd like some more information on that." So I gave them my formulas.

In 1982, I received my Masters in Nutrition from the University of Bridgeport, in Connecticut. And I kept on taking more and more courses in alternative healing. The more I studied, the more I realized that the new form of holistic dentistry I was envisioning was the only way to practice.

I began to involve myself in more holistic techniques. I had mostly given up on the methods used by my more mainstream colleagues. Of course, if a patient needed an antibiotic or some other drug, I would not hesitate if that was the best course of treatment.

I was now doing nonsurgical periodontal work—using herbs, homeopathic remedies, vitamins, and minerals—and was placing greater emphasis on nutrition. My patients thrived—and I became convinced that a healthy diet, exercise, reduced stress levels, and even prayer would restore the entire body to a healthy, vibrant state.

Today, I feel fortunate to be practicing holistic dentistry. I enjoy helping every patient avoid tooth and gum disease, and to use only nontoxic materials, in a noninvasive manner.

And my wish, in writing this book, is to enlighten every reader about the wonderful natural techniques now available to create perfect total health.

And that's just the beginning!

Here's to a healthier, happier you—

Dr. Victor Zeines
New York City
February 2000

PART
ONE

What *Is* Holistic Dentistry?

Now that you know how I got started in holistic dentistry, let's find out what this specialty is all about and what to expect in the pages ahead.

Perhaps the best way for me to begin is by making a few generalizations about holistic dentists. Not that they are all alike—far from it. Many have strong differences of opinion about their work, and like all dentists, some specialize in specific areas, from preventing cavities to reconstruction dentistry.

However, no matter what their differences may be, holistic dentists will certainly agree that the condition of your mouth reveals a lot about the overall state of your health. We recognize that your dental symptoms may be the result of an imbalance elsewhere in your body—and it's our job to find out exactly where and why.

The opposite is also true. Symptoms elsewhere in your body actually may be caused by problems in your mouth. There's plenty of research to suggest that harmful bacteria travel through the bloodstream to the heart, brain, and elsewhere, and cause problems wherever they land.

For too many years, conventional dentistry has focused on yanking deteriorated teeth or stuffing fillings filled with toxic materials—like mercury—without worrying about the aftermath or the underlying causes of the problem.

Holistic dentists, on the other hand, are always looking for the *underlying* causes of tooth and gum decay. They want to make certain that the problem does not recur.

And you may be surprised at the time and effort they are willing to devote to this task. In fact, they consider finding the cause of a symptom more important than the symptom itself.

Holistic dentists also try to minimize invasive treatment of the teeth and gums, an approach that endears us to our patients. For example, many conventional periodontists love one technique that their patients hate: They like to cut away infected tissue.

In contrast, I treat gum problems highly successfully with herbal rinses, good oral care, supplements, and through a healthy diet. The nutritional approach also addresses the underlying problem of what caused the gum disease in the first place. Gum disease should be considered more of a symptom than an actual problem. It is a symptom of excess acidity in the body.

I will only resort to surgery, antibiotics, and other drugs if the natural approaches I suggest don't do the trick. I certainly am not going to suggest that all periodontal surgery is unnecessary, only that gentler, natural solutions should be tried before a dentist resorts to radical invasive therapy.

This leads to another cardinal principle of holistic dentistry. We believe you need to give the body a chance to heal itself, and that is achieved by strengthening the immune system, the cornerstone of my practice.

In this book, I will share with you much of what I know. There is far more to dentistry than just getting X rays and fillings. I want you to become aware of the most painless, inexpensive, and effective ways to get that bright smile back on your face, and your mouth restored to full function.

For many dental patients, the most important advancement in dentistry has been anesthesia. I want to introduce you to even bigger changes—the use of herbs, vitamins, minerals, and techniques such as kinesiology, magnet therapy, and much more—in the field of dentistry.

In Part One, you will learn how best to avoid dental problems,

ne surprising information about what can cause oral disorders such
riodontal disease—stress is high on that list—and the most nat-
treatments available for such problems.

ot a toothache? The pain, and maybe even its cause, can be re-
l through herbs and homeopathic remedies. You will learn exactly
h herbs are best for you, and how to use homeopathy to improve
your health.

We will also be looking at diseases elsewhere in the body, and
learning how symptoms that appear in your mouth—like the discoloration of the tongue—can serve as an early warning to you that something is wrong. A visit to the dentist, in fact, may save you from a heart
attack!

You will also learn all about acidity in the mouth—a prime cause
of harmful bacterial infection—and what you can do about it.

Acidity is usually caused by too much sugar, dairy products, and
animal fats in your diet instead of plenty of fresh fruits and vegetables.
The more acid your body liquids become, the happier the bacteria that
cause tooth decay and gum disease.

I will give you a diet to change all this, and also explain how vitamins, minerals, and antioxidants can help you normalize your acid environment. You will also learn how to cleanse your body of toxins
before you even begin this new diet.

There are many controversies in the dental industry—from the potential hazards of fillings containing mercury, to the pros and cons of
fluoridation. Even the way root canal surgery is done is open to debate.
In this book, you will get all the facts about these controversies so that
you can make up your own mind.

In Part Two, I will share with you many of my treatments for a variety of dental problems—from gum disease to bad breath. I also talk
about "energy dentistry"—the use of techniques such as magnets, kinesiology, laser technology, and much more.

Believe it or not, in 1998 an estimated 60 million root canals were
performed. I find this shocking, because I consider root canal problems almost as dangerous as mercury fillings. In fact, I devote an entire
chapter to root canals—and why you should avoid them when possible.

I also go into some depth about cavitations—holes in the jaw that don't heal properly after a tooth is pulled. If your dentist is getting ready to pull that tooth, read this chapter carefully to avoid later problems after the extraction.

Much is being written nowadays about the potential dangers of amalgams. Why? Because mercury can wind up in body tissue and result in everything from birth defects to brain damage. Yet, amalgam fillings are still being used by many American dentists because the American Dental Society has not taken a strong stand against it, as have other health groups in countries like Sweden, Denmark, and Germany.

If you have mercury in your mouth—and which of us doesn't?—you will learn what you can do to remedy this problem, including how to detox from this and any other harmful metals that may be lodged in your body. As a holistic dentist, I'm not happy about the idea of putting anything metallic in a person's mouth—from bridges to implants.

Even if you currently have no major dental problems, this book will be of enormous value to you. Prevention is always the key to good health, and what you learn here will help keep your smile bright and your gums healthy.

So, finally, what is holistic dentistry? It is largely a matter of philosophy—the way your practitioner views dental health. A holistic dentist realizes that your oral health intimately affects, and is affected by, your physical health and vice versa.

A holistic dentist follows the Hippocratic ethic of "do no harm," and uses nontoxic methods and noninvasive techniques whenever possible.

Holistic health means taking a look at the entire body, finding out what the problems are, and changing the body from the teeth to the toes so that it can be a healthier place for you to inhabit.

My mission is to use as many treatment modalities that are natural. I view myself as part of a growing movement away from traditional drug therapies and treating the body as a separate entity.

For example, whenever I am lecturing to a group of dentists, the main concept that I try to get across is that the mouth is part of the whole body. We are not just "fixing teeth."

Repairing damaged or diseased tissue is only *part* of our job—the part that most dentists do quite well. Finding out why this damage is occurring is the aspect that is often sorely lacking in my profession.

So read on! Learn how to make the right choices to avoid unnecessary surgery and discover new ways to keep your mouth healthy. Let this book help you make lifestyle changes that will afford you the dental and physical health you so richly deserve.

CHOOSING A HOLISTIC DENTIST

Before selecting a holistic dentist, learn more about his or her attitude toward natural dental care. The following are some questions you may wish to consider asking on your first visit:

1. "Do you use a thyroid shield when taking x-rays?" (The thyroid gland is sensitive to radiation, and the effects can be serious.)
2. "Does your hygienist simply describe brushing and flossing, or does she actually teach you?" (A hands-on approach should be a cornerstone of your dentist's practice.)
3. "Do you use vitamin E and coenzyme Q-10 (you can read about these on page 63) to heal gums?" (Is the answer a knowledgeable one? Nutrition, after all, is a vital concept in holistic medical care.)
4. "Would you suggest a homeopathic remedy after today's treatment?" (Homeopathy plays an important role in holistic dentistry [see Chapter 9], and if your holistic dentist knows nothing about homeopathy, consider finding another one.)
5. "Do you know any holistic medical doctors?" (It is important that your dentist work cooperatively with such a doctor when dental problems have origins other than in the mouth.)
6. "After examining my mouth, do you discuss the possible causes of my problems during the first visit or two—or do you tell me how many cavities I have and then get to work?" (If it's the latter, you

have a dentist who is not treating you like an intelligent partner.)

7. "Will you discuss the color of my tongue? Do you use kinesiology to test the temporomandibular joint (TMJ)?" For details, see chapter 2.

8. Do you use mercury fillings?

9. Do you detox patients when removing mercury?

CHAPTER 2

Welcome to My Office

Come on in!

This is probably your first visit to a holistic dentist's office, so let me first give you an overall view about exactly what goes on here. Then we'll examine each of the steps in a little more detail. In the process, I'm going to show you some techniques for checking out the condition of your own dental health.

Let me begin by saying that a good holistic dentist, like a good conventional dentist, uses sterile instruments and the latest and best equipment. Holistic dentists, however, seem to be fond of more gizmos than their more conservative colleagues.

So feel free to look around. In my office you'll find all kinds of neat stuff—everything from a digital radiograph and ultra-cam intra-oval camera, which allows you to see what your tooth looks like but is a safer alternative to those x-rays—to trays of vitamins, minerals, and homeopathic remedies.

Take a seat. The first thing I want to know about you has nothing to do with your teeth or gums, but, rather, about your general health. I'll take a look at both your medical and dental records, and ask you some questions.

After I have formed an impression of your general health, I'll examine your left and right temporomandibular joints (TMJs). These are the joints connecting your upper and lower jawbones, and they are located on either side of your face, near your ears.

I adhere to many of the teachings of Oriental medicine. This ancient and time-honored tradition considers these joints to be one of the major energy points of the body.

Great care must be taken to make certain that these joints are in proper alignment in order to avoid possible problems not only with the teeth—but with the neck, shoulders, arms, and back, as well.

Even before I examine your mouth, the result of this simple and painless TMJ test will give me the first indication if there are any special problems elsewhere in the body that may need attention.

If your TMJs are out of whack, it can have a wide-ranging effect on the total state of your body—from headaches to stress. We'll be talking a lot more about TMJs later on, and even explain how you can conduct your own test.

Next, let me examine you for any evidence of oral cancer. I'll be looking for lumps and lesions and other physical signs. This will be followed by a tongue diagnosis to check for the presence of any general health problems.

Checking the tongue is a very important part of my examination. One of the basic concepts of holistic dentistry is that the mouth is an indicator of the state of health of the body.

Tissue changes, including tongue discoloration, all play a part in diagnosis and treatment plan. Doctors, by the way, have been checking the tongue going way back into Chinese history. If you want to know how your tongue rates on the health scale, you'll find a chart later in this chapter that will reveal this information.

Finally, using state-of-the-art x-ray equipment, I will now look at your teeth, searching for signs of tooth decay. When I finish, I'll review your medical history to investigate possible connections between any dental problems and illnesses in other parts of your body. If I detect a medical problem outside the scope of dentistry, I will recommend that you see a physician for diagnosis and treatment.

That's the general procedure. Now let's take a look at it in some more detail:

General Health Appraisal

One of the first things I do when you walk into my office is observe the shape of your body, the look of your skin, the way you move, talk, and respond. All of these give me an overview of your general state of health. Do your eyes show any redness or yellowness? (Yellowness might indicate a liver problem.)

Are your eyes dull or bright? The condition of your fingernails also says a lot about your health. Are your nails bitten? Are they broken? (Frequent nail breaking usually means that you have a mineral deficiency.) To some extent, we all make these observations when we meet people. We notice how great someone's hair or complexion looks—or doesn't.

A psychiatrist friend once told me that he often relied on the condition of a female patient's hair to gauge her state of health. When her hair looked dry, lifeless, and uncared for, chances were the patient was depressed.

On the other hand, when his patient arrived with glistening, well-tended tresses, the good doctor said, "Ah, I see you are feeling better."

"How did you know?" the patient would inevitably ask, astonished at the doctor's insight.

Temporomandibular Joint (TMJ) Checkup

To check TMJ alignment, I ask the patient to place his or her index fingers on either side of the head, just in front of the ears. I then have the patient open and close the mouth.

The joint on each side of the head that you feel moving backward and forward as you do so, is your TMJ. If you hear a clicking sound as you open and close your mouth, this generally means that the TMJ is not in its proper position and may need some adjustment.

When the jaw, or mandible, is not in proper alignment, many of the muscles of the head and neck try to compensate for this and develop their own source of tension. The back muscles are similarly affected.

This joint can be a source of stress that gets worse during periods of sleep, when the body is trying to rest or recover from work. The continuing stress from an improperly functioning jawbone can actually speed up the aging process!

If you get head or neck aches with some frequency, you may have a TMJ problem. A TMJ problem can also be responsible for shoulder pain, earache, tinnitus, blurred vision, vertigo, and jaw spasms.

When your jaws close, your teeth should meet and fit together evenly. If the cusp or biting edge of one tooth does not fit because it is too high or out of position, your teeth may no longer meet comfortably together.

This can be a consequence of dental work or of a tooth changing position. Your bite (occlusion) is now uneven. This new, uncomfortable closure is likely to cause stress. Without being aware of it, you may begin clenching your teeth and jaws, and grinding your teeth.

This causes the nerves in the teeth and roots to become pinched, which adds even more stress. Grinding can also loosen teeth, opening pockets between the tooth and gum for harmful bacteria to penetrate.

Dentists have a number of solutions to TMJ problems. A dental appliance worn at night can prevent grinding while you are asleep. Filing down a raised cusp may restore your bite to its natural fit. Kinesiology is also a valuable tool.

I find kinesiological tests to be one of the best ways of checking the health of this joint. According to Chinese medicine, the TMJ is one of the main balancing points of the body, and much of the body's energy flows through this area.

Kinesiology lets me know if the energy is flowing in a healthy manner. If it is, I know the body is in balance. In Chapter 19, we will discuss how kinesiology works in much greater detail.

The word *kinesiology* (or *kinetics*) comes from the study of muscle and joint movements. This method of measuring the body's energy field was developed in 1964 by George Goodheart.

KINESIOLOGY SELF-TEST

You can try this simple kinesiology test with a friend. Hold one arm out so that it is parallel to the floor. Have a friend gently press down on the hand that is extended, and notice the amount of strength you need to resist the downward motion.

Then hold sugar or tobacco in your other, unextended hand, while your friend gently presses down again on the hand that is extended. If you are like most people, you will notice that the strength you need to keep your hand in position is much greater than before. This means that the substance you are holding has caused some kind of weakness in your body.

When something that can cause you harm enters your energy field—such as the example of sugar or tobacco given above—it can adversely affect your energy and your health. This disruption will show in the reaction of your muscles during a kinesiology test.

Of all the people I have tested this way, more than 90 percent have some sort of malposition of the TMJ joint. This is not surprising when you consider the amount of stress the average person is under, and the amount of teeth clenching and grinding caused by stress.

Once TMJ testing is completed, I make a simple adjustment. I take the jaw and with both hands on the sides of the head I gently push the jaw down and forward. This will bring the jaw into balance and hopefully help with other physical problems.

Afterwards, many of my patients report that their breathing is better, they have more energy, or they feel more relaxed. Neck or back aches or pains are either gone or lessened. This testing is important for another reason.

Many people have restorations (fillings or crowns) that are not positioned properly. After a test and adjustment, such teeth tend to realign slightly in a more proper manner.

Nutritional Therapy for TMJ

Some people who suffer from TMJ problems may be hypoglycemic, a condition that is often caused by low blood sugar. This means that the body is not getting enough calcium, leading to an eroding of the teeth, which then leads to the clenching or grinding of teeth.

The following supplements may be helpful for such a nutritional deficiency. Also, avoid eating a high-protein breakfast (such as eggs) as well as refined sugar, caffeine, and alcohol.

Magnesium, 1000 mg (helps muscle metabolism)
Calcium, 500 mg (helps muscle metabolism)
Manganese (helps ligaments heal)
Vitamin B-complex (relieves stress)
Vitamin C (antiinflammation)
L-phenylalanine (pain relief, mood improvement)
Coenzyme Q10 (healing energy)
Omega fatty acids
Calming herbs, such as valerian root, chamomile, skull-cap, and passion flower

Oral Cancer Checkup

Oral cancer affects approximately 30,000 Americans each year. On average, only 50 percent of those with the disease survive five years. Early detection can increase this survival rate to 76 percent. Early warning signs in the mouth are easy to see or feel. Symptoms may include:

Red or white lesions in the mouth
Lump in the throat
Thickening or lump in the oral lining
Tongue numbness
Ear pain
Tooth pain (sometimes)

In an oral cancer checkup, the dentist carefully checks your lips, cheeks, tongue, and the tissue beneath your tongue. The hard and soft palate are also checked. The glands under the jaw are felt and any abnormalities noted.

Tongue Diagnosis

Tongue diagnosis has been used in Chinese medicine for more than two thousand years. Over 280 diseases can be diagnosed through proper use of this method.

Remember when you were a kid? What was the first thing that your doctor did when you visited him or he made a house call? That's right—he made you stick out your tongue! Now you know where Western doctors got the idea.

The physician then checked your tongue color for an indication of your general state of health. For example, the tongue of someone with a bad cold or the flu will have a white coating, revealing that toxins are being released from the body.

In my practice, it's not unusual for me to see yellow, yellow-green, gray, or brownish-gray tongues. I then explain to my patient that the condition of the tongue suggests there may be a problem elsewhere in their body that needs correction, and that the problem is not really with the tooth or gums.

All that explanation is not as effective as giving the patient a mirror and letting him or her have a look at the color of the tongue. They'll say something like, "Oh, my tongue looks yellowish, but I thought it was supposed to be pink?" And I'll say, "Yes, it's supposed to be pink."

In fact, I remember one particular patient—Michael—who was very hard to convince. He came into my office because of a problem with bleeding gums. Michael was overweight and I did a diet analysis with him. He saw what was going on with his body, but he really wasn't interested in changing his lifestyle.

When I held the mirror up to his face and had him stick his tongue out, he finally got the message. Michael saw that his tongue was a bright yellow color.

He asked, "What does it mean, that my tongue is so yellow?" I said, "It means that your gallbladder may not be functioning properly." Until then he didn't believe me. But he *did* believe what he saw in the mirror.

Michael went on a diet, and three or four weeks later you could see the change in his tongue. In fact, he called me in a panic. He said, "Doctor, now my tongue is white!"

I laughed. Michael didn't know this was good news, but the white color told me that toxins were being released. I asked, "Are you losing weight?"

He said, "Yes, and I have a lot more energy and my headaches are gone."

Another three weeks passed. Not only were his headaches gone, but his gums were bleeding less. Michael said he was feeling better than ever and his tongue had turned pink.

Okay, put down the book for a moment. Take a look at your tongue in a mirror. What is its color? Are there indentations or cracks? A healthy tongue is pink and has no indentations or cracks on the surface. Consult the following chart to find out how healthy your tongue might be.

If your tongue shows any of these conditions, relax, don't panic. This is an early warning to begin paying attention to a deficiency in your body, and get the problem corrected.

When I find a tongue that's signaling for help, I suggest that my

Tongue Condition	Indicative of
Yellowish or yellow-green	Liver or gallbladder problems
Gray or brownish-gray	Stomach or intestinal problems
White	Body releasing toxins
A border, with the edges showing the teeth outlines	Mineral deficiency
Indentations or cracks on the surface	Vitamin deficiency

patient begin a liver-gallbladder flush combined with a body-cleansing diet. You'll get all the details of these two cleanses on pages 40, 41.

Teeth Examination

In my initial consultation, I use an ultra-cam intra-oval camera, which allows both my patients and me to instantly view their teeth on a monitor.

During this stage of the examination, I note restorations, missing or unerupted teeth, and problems such as decayed, cracked, or broken teeth. (We will look more closely at the problems of teeth in the following chapters.)

I then use a digital radiograph to take x-rays. While I am not a big fan of x-rays, they are often essential because they can show 50 percent more areas of decay than a visual examination.

X-rays also show the internal workings of the tooth, including the nerves and supporting structures such as bone and the periodontal ligaments. In spite of the risk of cancer-causing radiation and generation of free radicals inherent in x-rays, their benefits more than justify their careful use on an infrequent number of occasions.

When you have dental x-rays taken, make sure that your dentist is using a digital radiographic unit. Having used digital units for some time, I find them to be superior to conventional radiographs.

With a digital radiograph, I can enlarge areas that seem suspicious and colorize pictures so that more information can be obtained from light differences. A digital picture appears instantly.

Also, with a digital radiograph, should a picture be required in the course of a procedure, there's never any delay while waiting for film to be developed. Digital machines also decrease your exposure to radiation by 90 percent, because they use a sensor and computer instead of x-ray film. Much less radiation is needed for a sensor than film.

How many x-rays should be taken? The answer to that question depends on how long ago it's been since you last had dental x-rays, and the number you had taken at that time.

The general condition of your mouth is another factor that would help me decide how many and which pictures I need. For example, someone forty-five years old, with three fillings received at the age of fourteen, does not need as many pictures as someone the same age with a mouth full of restorations and ongoing decay. Here are some recommendations:

- A full set of x-rays should not be taken more than once in three years.
- Pregnant women should avoid x-rays.
- Lead shielding must be worn when x-rays are being taken.
- A thyroid shield should also be used. Your thyroid gland is sensitive to radiation.

If your dentist suggests that x-rays will be taken on your next visit, I'd suggest that you head over to your nearest health food store. Pick up the following supplements, which can offer you some protection against x-rays because they work chiefly as antioxidants and precancer suppressants. Start taking them a few days before your next appointment, and continue taking them for at least two days after the visit. Follow the instructions on the labels for how many of these supplements you should take and when.

Beta-carotene plus entire carotene complex, 5000 IU
Pycnogenol ®, 100 mg
Coenzyme Q10, 100 mg
Vitamin E, mixed tocopherols, 400 IU
Selenium, 150 mcg
Vitamin C, 500 mg, four times a day

Once your examination is over, should you need some kind of dental work, then it's time to discuss all the options. I want you to become my partner when deciding what kind of treatment is right for you.

I am not the kind of dentist who simply tells you how many cavities you have and then gets ready to go to work. The word "doctor" derives from the Latin word "teacher," and that's what I'm here to do.

I also want us to talk about how this problem got started in the first place. This is the only way that both of us will learn from this experience. It is through understanding your body and what needs to be done to heal it that you will grow into new ways of thinking and prevent future dental problems.

CHAPTER 3

Relax, It's Not Going to Hurt

One of the main problems I have had being a dentist is dealing with fear—not mine, but seeing someone looking at me for the first time with an expression of naked terror on his or her face.

I always ask, "How did you get my number?" "Oh, so and so recommended you," the patient will reply. "They said you were great and very gentle. The work was good and you didn't hurt."

So why do you have the same look on your face that I would associate with receiving a box of live rattlesnakes?

As a child, I, too, was always afraid of dentists. Going to the dentist was the worst! I would hold on to the dentist's chair with both hands and hope the dentist didn't notice how badly I was sweating. So I do understand how my patients may feel. But guess what? In my office you don't need to be afraid. I promise that I'm not going to hurt you!

As a holistic dentist, I'm a very caring person. If I need to give you an injection, my goal is to make that injection as painless as possible, and that is easily done. I give you my word on that. So what exactly are you afraid of?

If I may speak as a former psychotherapist, I believe that one reason for such fear is that when you open your mouth, you are in a very real way opening yourself and trusting that vulnerable part of your body to another human being.

That has been one of the problems in our society—fear of vulnerability—although I think that nowadays that attitude is slowly changing. We are learning that it is okay to be vulnerable in front of others. Real men do cry!

Another reason some patients experience fear is that just sitting in the dental chair brings up old childhood traumas that they may not even be consciously aware of. I've had many patients over the years tell me that they are terrified, despite my having given them anesthesia before, and performing a painless procedure.

Even though they are aware that this is a painless procedure, they still break out in a cold sweat. Why? What is actually causing this fear? Perhaps it's an old memory of childhood visits to dentists now being replayed on an unconscious level.

Fear of violation may be another reason. Some patients experience a dentist's hands in their mouths as such a violation. I can understand how it feels.

When I was studying acupuncture, I had no trouble sticking those little needles into somebody else's skin. But I found it very hard to have acupuncture done to me.

Generally, needles do not bother me. But there is something about the way acupuncture changes my energy field (even though it is helping me) that I find hard to take. It's a violation of sorts. So you see, even dentists can have the same anxieties as you do.

When I give an injection, I do it so gently that the feeling of being violated is either markedly reduced or removed. I also utilize homeopathic and essential oil applications, all designed to make you feel much more at ease in the dentist's chair.

If you are one of those patients who is afraid of dentists, I'd suggest that one way to rid yourself of that fear is by talking about it with your practitioner. Let him or her know, for example, that you are terrified of injections.

Most dentists will be happy to talk to you about their procedure with a needle, and I believe this exchange will help to lessen your fears. If nothing else, you've established a more open doctor-patient relationship.

It may also help knowing that there are some topical anesthetics which so anesthetize the skin, the needle is not even felt. I tend to favor these substances when they are needed, although in most cases just proceeding gently and carefully is an equally effective pain-free approach.

If you're the anxious type, one technique that you may find to be quite effective in helping to control your anxiety is visualization. Visualization is a way of conjuring up beautiful and peaceful thoughts in your mind's eye.

If you are getting anesthesia or some other kind of treatment, instead of thinking fearful thoughts, try to concentrate on the colors pink or green. Visualize, for example, a green field where thousands of pink lilies are growing.

Pink is known for its soothing effect and is often used to calm patients. Green is also well known for its calming effect. You might also want to visualize a clear blue sky in the area of the injection.

Blue is a color that is often associated with healing. Taking deep slow breaths when the anesthesia is given also helps. It's surprising how many people hold their breath when they get apprehensive. Letting go and relaxing your body through deep slow breathing and color visualizations will go a long way to allay your anxieties.

Many of my patients ask for Valium or gas to help cope with their fear and anxiety. I try to avoid using either substance. When you take Valium or are given nitrous oxide, in a very real way you are no longer with your dentist.

"So?" you might ask. "What's wrong with that?" The problem as I see it is that you never get to experience what is actually going on, and as a result, that fear will never leave you. You'll return time after time with the same set of anxieties.

I am concerned that if you get into such an avoidance mode, you will also avoid other problems in your mouth or the rest of your body. Do you remember seeing dragons in your yard as a child? You would tell your mother all about it and she would say, "Pay no attention and it will go away."

In real life, however, dental problems will not go away if you ignore them. And neither will your fears if you don't deal with them without sedatives or other substances. The only way you can successfully banish the dragon is by confronting it. By the way, a dragon has never been spotted in my dental office!

Okay, you can handle the anesthetic, but it's the noise of the drill that makes you want to run for the hills. Yes, I wish I or someone else had invented a silent drill. Aside from the money I would have earned, I would have had the gratitude of every dental patient in the world.

But there are ways to cope with such noise. For example, earplugs can be very helpful. This is a very practical way to make your visit a little less stressful.

Earphones plugged into a tape player can provide you with a very relaxing and stress-reducing experience. Many of my patients do just that. They bring their own tape or CD player, and I very much encourage that.

Another thing you might do is use an alpha wave generator. This is a device that looks like a large pair of goggles. You place these goggles over your eyes, and they emit a pulsating light in which one of two things happen:

1. You zone out as your brain begins to generate alpha waves and don't hear the drill.
2. You get so bored with these pulsations, that you take the goggles off and look forward to hearing the drill and participating in your dental experience.

What I really want to make you understand is that your dental visit does not have to be associated with fear of pain. It's easy enough to make your dental visit stress free.

While it's true that you may never want to see your dentist except, perhaps, on social occasions, using some of these techniques will ensure that your dental visit can become a pleasant experience.

CHAPTER 4

Knocking Out Those Pesky Bacteria

A strong immune system means healthy teeth and gums. In my practice, I have discovered that many dental problems have their origins in the body's inability to function properly.

When your immune system is not functioning properly, your resistance to bacteria is low, and what started out as tooth decay or periodontal disease can, according to some new research, result in everything from heart attacks and strokes to diabetes.

An improper diet, for example, can cause an imbalance in the calcium-phosphorus ratio in the mouth and allow harmful bacteria to grow. Too much food containing phosphorus creates an acidic environment in the mouth, which is paradise for harmful bacteria.

Once the gums are infected, the bacteria continues to spread until it invades and destroys the bone that supports the teeth. If not treated in time, big problems can develop—not only in the oral cavity, but elsewhere in the body as well.

Stress is another culprit that can lead to periodontal disease. Excessive amounts of stress drain your immune system of vital minerals and vitamins, depleting your immune system.

Stress also interferes with the production of saliva, which not only is vital for maintaining lubrication in the mouth, but has bacteria-fighting properties. So if you're not eating right or are leading a high-stress lifestyle, you may find yourself welcoming unwanted bacteria into your mouth.

An acidic environment in the mouth caused by too many sweets, fat, and dairy can also strip tooth enamel of its minerals, thus weakening that tooth and making it more vulnerable to attack by bacteria.

We'll be talking more about acid and alkaline foods later on, and I will even give you a shopping list of foods that can vastly improve your oral health. In addition, you'll learn how to test yourself to see exactly how much acid there is in your mouth.

Right now, you need to remember that foods rich in calcium and magnesium are good for your teeth and gums. Green leafy vegetables and bananas are excellent sources for these minerals.

Some years ago, when author and humorist Lewis Grizzard died of heart disease at the age of forty-seven, one doctor who consulted on the case made an unusual observation.

"He had bad teeth," Atlanta oral surgeon Thomas Boc told USA Today. "He wouldn't floss, he wouldn't brush. He was a classic example of somebody whose chronic dental infection led to chronic heart disease, valve failure and ultimately death."

Sound far-fetched? Not if you've been practicing holistic dentistry for as long as I have. Over the years I have observed a direct correlation between gum disease and bacterial infection elsewhere in the body.

There is, today, growing clinical evidence that even small infections in your mouth may be a contributing factor to everything from arterial plaque, diabetes, and stroke, to preterm births.

If you are healthy, the bad bacteria in your mouth (and they're always present) are prevented from spreading by your saliva, which contains germ-killing properties. But if your immune system is bent out of shape, watch out! Those pesky critters will take full advantage of you.

Eating poorly, not exercising regularly, and allowing stress to run your life can all contribute to an impaired immune system and, ultimately, dental infection. And once harmful bacteria gain a foothold in your mouth, they tend to breed and spread faster than rabbits.

Many dentists and other physicians believe that these bacteria first attack the bones and gums in the mouth, and then continue to march along the bloodstream and attack us where we are most vulnerable. They enter our bloodstream through small cracks in the gums which appear when we suffer from periodontal disease.

Big Plaque Attack

I tend to agree with this theory. I believe that the same things that are happening in your mouth are most likely happening to the rest of your body! That sticky plaque you brush off your teeth and the plaque that builds up inside the arteries seem to be similar. Arteriosclerotic plaque is predominantly a buildup of calcium—just like the mouth.

So if you've got a severe case of plaque, beware! Unless you take steps to remedy the situation, you may be a candidate for heart disease. How's that as an excellent reason to go out right now and buy some floss?

You *Are* What You Eat

Researchers are also making a link between severe cases of gum disease and diabetes, since both problems are related to blood sugars in the body.

Dr. Christopher Saudek, a diabetes specialist at Johns Hopkins University in Maryland, recently told an interviewer that "people with diabetes should be careful to keep their gums healthy." He worried that gum disease is evidence of a poorly working immune system, making it easier for bacteria from the mouth to spread.

While this research is still controversial, it is well known that periodontal disease can worsen diabetes. The bacterial infection that is causing the gum disease seems to make insulin work less efficiently.

In my practice I see a lot of patients who are prediabetic because of problems with too much sugar. That's why one of the first things I do with my new patients is to have them do a diet analysis. It's a real wakeup call when these people see what they're eating. You'd be absolutely amazed at how much sugar there is in processed foods.

Many of my patients who are prediabetic are malnourished. One case I especially remember is Sally. She came into my office one day and I discovered that she was a borderline diabetic.

"My diet is good," she told me.

"That's kind of hard for me to accept because your mouth is bleeding," I replied. "Your gums are bleeding every time you brush your teeth. Something's got to be wrong."

Sally looked at me for a few moments, letting that register.

"How are your stress levels?" I asked her.

"High," she replied.

Sally kept resisting my efforts to talk to her about diet and nutrition, promising instead to quit her job of twenty years in order to reduce her stress. I told her that might be a good idea, but we still needed to talk about proper nutrition.

Finally, Sally allowed me to do a diet analysis. Her diet was what was considered the great American diet in the 1950s. It consisted of breakfast with toast, a lot of butter, and coffee with lots of cream and sugar.

For lunch, she ate a sandwich made of some kind of processed meat, while for dinner Sally consumed lots of meat, which she liked to eat late at night—around nine or ten o'clock.

With the four or five cups of coffee with sugar that she drank between meals, I realized that Sally was eating a good half pound of sugar each day.

I told Sally that all that sugar in her body was a perfect breeding ground for bacteria. Sugar is nothing but a carbohydrate glue that bacteria like to feed on. It was creating an environment in which her mouth chemistry was changing. The result was certain to be a serious case of gum disease and, possibly, diabetes down the line.

Sally changed her diet. In a couple of weeks her gums were no longer bleeding. The condition simply vanished. Coming to see me may have also prevented her from becoming a victim of diabetes.

The biggest lesson here is that all of this could have been prevented in the first place if Sally had paid more attention to what she was eating and drinking.

There is an old saying: "You are what you eat." More than 60 percent of our population is overweight because they simply don't care what kinds of food they eat. What we need to do is to start looking at wholesome, natural, inexpensive ways to stay healthy and enjoy a better quality of life.

The Long and Winding Road

There are more than 400 species of bacteria that live in your mouth—and you thought it was crowded on the subways!

Many of these bacteria are beneficial. Others are simply neutral. Some, however, are killer bacteria that many scientists believe travel through the bloodstream from teeth to toes.

Let's take a brief look at the suspected links between gum disease and the long, winding road to other medical problems.

1. Heart Disease

Who, for example, would have thought that a visit to your dentist's office could protect your heart? But according to recent studies, there is a heart-gums connection. Untreated bleeding gums stemming from either gingivitis or periondontis appear to be precursors to various cardiovascular problems.

According to one study conducted by the University of Buffalo, the same bacteria causing those gum problems end up either directly infecting your heart arteries or somehow causing other blockages.

Another study—this one done in 1998 at the University of Minnesota—showed that by injecting rabbits with tooth plaque bacteria, the same bacteria caused blood clots which led to heart attacks.

In a recent article in the *Vegetarian Times*, Eugene J. Whitacker, an associate professor of dentistry at Temple University, said that "at least 36 million Americans have some form of destructive periodontal disease."

The professor concluded that "these people may be at an increased risk of getting heart disease and stroke if the plaque bacteria from their mouths get into the bloodstream."

The dentist also noted that people under the age of fifty seem to be especially vulnerable to heart attacks linked to oral infection.

2. Stroke

If your gums are infected, you triple your risk of having a stroke, according to a 1998 study of 166 stroke victims done at the University of Heidelberg in Germany.

In yet another study conducted at the University of Buffalo, researchers surveyed the health history of 9,982 people from twenty-five to seventy-five and found that the 35 percent with severe gum disease were twice as likely to have a stroke. They identified oral bacteria as the cause, explaining that these harmful microorganisms may travel on and cause fatty accumulations in the carotid arteries.

3. Premature, Low-Birthweight Babies

At the University of Alabama, Researcher Marjorie Jeffcoat recently discovered that among 120 women in rural Alabama, those with dental infections were three times more likely to have premature, low-birthweight babies than women with healthy teeth and gums.

4. Bronchitis, Pneumonia, and Emphysema

Clinical studies have shown that chronic bronchitis, emphysema, and other respiratory ailments all worsened when harmful oral bacteria were inhaled. When such bacteria were breathed into the lungs, and the immune system could not overcome them, bacterial pneumonia resulted.

5. Vision Impairment

Russian-American dentist Edward Hutton described in an article how a twenty-three-year-old patient told him that she had been in a wheelchair since she was thirteen. Her double vision was so severe, she couldn't stand or walk unaided.

Dr. Hutton learned that six months before her vision had deteriorated, two of the young woman's upper teeth had been pulled for orthodontic treatment.

"Two pockets of infection formed where the teeth had been pulled," the dentist said. "The surrounding teeth exerted pressure on these infected pockets and forced them against the nerve. That pressure on the nerve is what caused the double vision."

As Dr. Hutton drained the infected pockets, the patient suddenly exclaimed, "I can see!"

When the procedure was over, "She got up from the chair and walked away unaided for the first time in ten years," Dr. Hutton explained. "There were tears in the eyes of everyone in the room."

Now able to read once more, the young woman completed high school and is presently attending college.

6. Implant Infections

Researchers also suspect that bacteria traveling from the mouth through the bloodstream may be responsible for infections around artificial heart valves, artificial joints, or other synthetic implants. If you have any type of implant and are anticipating dental treatment, it is recommended by dentists that you take antibiotics before beginning your treatment.

7. Pain, Pain, Go Away

Over the years, patients have come into my office with a variety of complaints pertaining to pain, from headaches to ear and neck problems.

Often, these problems are the result of oral infections. I remember one patient who came in and complained to me about tinnitus, or a ringing in his ears.

For Robert, a thirty-five-year-old car salesman, this had been a chronic problem for many years—until I replaced his mercury fillings and refilled his teeth with nontoxic substances called composite fillings, which will be discussed later. The only ringing my patient heard from that day on was the sound of the cash register for the cars he sold!

I thought that was the end of his dental problems until two

Relationships Between Teeth and Other Areas of the Body

Tooth	SENSE ORGANS	Joints	VERTEBRAE	ORGANS	ENDOCRINE GLANDS	OTHERS
R						
1	Inner Ear	Shoulder elbow; Hand ulnar foot plantar toes, sacroiliac joint	C7 T1 T5 T6 S1 S2	Heart; Duodenum	Ant. lobe of pituitary	CNS Psyche
2	Maxillary Sinus	Jaws; Front of knee	T11 T12 L1	Pancreas; Stomach	Para-thyroid	Mammary gland
3	Maxillary Sinus	Jaws; Front of knee	T11 T12 L1	Pancreas; Stomach	Thyroid	Mammary gland
4	Ethmoid Cell	Shoulder Elbow; Hand radial foot Big toe	C5 C6 C7 T3 T4 L4 L5	Lung; Large intestine	Thymus	
5	Ethmoid Cell	Shoulder Elbow; Hand radial foot Big toe	C5 C6 C7 T3 T4 L4 L5	Lung; Large intestine	Post. lobe of pituitary	
6	Eye	Hip; Foot	T9 T10	Liver; Gall-bladder	Post. lobe of pituitary	
7	Frontal Sinus	Back of knee; Sacrococcyx; Foot	L2 L3 S3 S4 S5 Coccyx	Kidney; Bladder Urogenital area	Pineal gland	
8	Frontal Sinus	Back of knee; Sacrococcyx; Foot		Kidney; Bladder Urogenital area	Pineal gland	
L						
9	Frontal Sinus	Back of knee; Sacrococcyx; Foot		Kidney; Bladder Urogenital area	Pineal gland	
10	Frontal Sinus	Back of knee; Sacrococcyx; Foot		Kidney; Bladder Urogenital area	Pineal gland	
11	Eye	Hip; Foot	T9 T10	Liver; Gall-bladder	Post. lobe of pituitary	
12	Ethmoid Cell	Shoulder Elbow; Hand radial foot Big toe	C5 C6 C7 T3 T4 L4 L5	Lung; Large intestine	Post. lobe of pituitary	
13	Ethmoid Cell	Shoulder Elbow; Hand radial foot Big toe	C5 C6 C7 T3 T4 L4 L5	Lung; Large intestine	Thymus	
14	Maxillary Sinus	Jaws; Front of knee	T11 T12 L1	Pancreas; Stomach	Thyroid	Mammary gland
15	Maxillary Sinus	Jaws; Front of knee	T11 T12 L1	Pancreas; Stomach	Para-thyroid	Mammary gland
16	Inner Ear	Shoulder elbow; Hand ulnar foot plantar toes, sacroiliac joint	C7 T1 T5 T6 S1 S2	Heart; Duodenum	Ant. lobe of pituitary	CNS Psyche

Tooth–organ correspondence chart (L = teeth 17–24, R = teeth 25–32)

Tooth	OTHERS	ENDOCRINE GLDS / TISSUE SYSTEMS	ORGANS	VERTEBRAE	JOINTS	SENSE ORGANS
17 (L)	Energy metabolism	Peripheral nerves	Ileum; Ileocecal region; Heart	C7; T1 T5 T6; S1 S2	Shoulder and elbow; Hand ulnar, Foot plantar, Toes. sacro-iliac joint	Ear
18		Arteries	Large intestine; Ileocecal region; Lung	C5 C6 C7; T3 T4; L4 L5	Shoulder and elbow; Hand radial, Foot, Big toe	Ethmoid cells
19	Mammary gland	Veins	Large intestine; Ileocecal region; Lung	C5 C6 C7; T3 T4; L4 L5	Hand radial, Foot, Big toe	Ethmoid cells
20	Mammary gland	Lymph vessels	Stomach Pylorus; Pancreas	T11; T12; L1	Front of knee; Jaws	Maxillary sinus
21		Gonad	Stomach Pylorus; Pancreas	T11; T12; L1	Front of knee; Jaws	
22		Gonad	Gall-bladder; Liver	T9; T10	Hip	Eye
23		Adrenal gld	Bladder Urogenital area; Kidney	L2 L3; S3 S4 S5; Coccyx	Back of knee; Foot	Frontal sinus
24		Adrenal gld	Bladder Urogenital area; Kidney	L2 L3; S3 S4 S5; Coccyx	Sacrococcyx; Foot	Frontal sinus
25 (R)		Adrenal gld	Bladder Urogenital area; Kidney	L2 L3; S3 S4 S5; Coccyx	Sacrococcyx; Foot	Frontal sinus
26		Adrenal gld	Bladder Urogenital area; Kidney	L2 L3; S3 S4 S5; Coccyx	Back of knee; Foot	Frontal sinus
27		Gonad	Gall-bladder; Liver	T9; T10	Hip	Eye
28		Gonad	Stomach Pylorus; Pancreas	T11; T12; L1	Front of knee; Jaws	
29	Mammary gland	Lymph vessels	Stomach Pylorus; Pancreas	T11; T12; L1	Front of knee; Jaws	Maxillary sinus
30	Mammary gland	Veins	Large intestine; Ileocecal region; Lung	C5 C6 C7; T3 T4; L4 L5	Hand radial, Foot, Big toe	Ethmoid cells
31		Arteries	Large intestine; Ileocecal region; Lung	C5 C6 C7; T3 T4; L4 L5	Shoulder and elbow; Hand radial, Foot, Big toe	Ethmoid cells
32 (R)	Energy metabolism	Peripheral nerves	Ileum; Ileocecal region; Heart	C7; T1 T5 T6; S1 S2	Shoulder and elbow; Hand ulnar, Foot plantar, Toes. sacro-iliac joint	Ear

months later, when I heard from Robert, again. This time he complained about pain in the back of his head. "I can't tell you how many doctors I've gone to, and it's still there," he said. "Could it be from cavitations?"

A cavitation, which we discuss more fully in Chapter 16, is essentially a hole in the jawbone, usually where a tooth has been removed and the bone cavity has not filled in properly.

They are a good medium for infections to grow in, creating a variety of other physical problems. Unfortunately, these cavitations do not generally show up on x-rays, so if the patient is not experiencing any pain, there is no real reason to look for them.

Robert, however, had guessed right. He had two cavitations—one on each side of his mouth—and I thoroughly cleaned both of them out. There were all kinds of debris there—pieces of leftover membrane and bits of dead bone material. His dentist obviously had not been too meticulous when removing the teeth.

I also treated the infections I found in both areas with herbs and other natural substances. To both my own and my patient's delight, Robert's head pain soon disappeared.

If you are experiencing unexplained chronic pain whether in the face, head, neck, or shoulders, and your doctor can't seem to get a handle on what is causing it, the cause may have something to do with those pesky bacteria.

If your doctor can't seem to find the source of the problem, it might not be a bad idea to talk to your dentist—especially if you have had molars or wisdom teeth extracted, or had a root canal done.

For a fascinating look at how the mouth and body are interrelated, consider the table on pages 32 and 33.

CHAPTER 5

The High Price of Convenience

Nowadays, we're seeing diseases such as cancer, heart disease, arthritis, chronic fatigue, and periodontal disease reaching epidemic proportions.

Is this so surprising, when each year the average American is exposed to fourteen pounds of food preservatives, additives, pesticides, and herbal residues?

In this chapter, we're going to look at the benefits of various detox programs—from a liver-gallbladder flush to an internal cleanse, which will allow the body to get rid of accumulated waste products, irritants, and toxins while restoring intestinal health.

But before we do so, let's try to determine where we went wrong. How did we human beings go from vegetarians who got plenty of good exercise foraging in the forests, to couch potatoes who thrive on diets of pizza and McDonald's?

Homo habilis, or "Handyman," appeared about 2.5 million years ago. He was the first of our ancestors to learn how to use tools, hammering on rocks to crack and form them into more useful shapes.

Our distant ancestors were under five feet tall and weighed less than a hundred pounds. These humanoids were scavengers, supplementing a vegetarian diet with meat from leftover predator kills, as well as insects. Grain was another food source in open country.

Their molars ground up small, hard objects, and their hinged jaws had the power and the side-to-side movement necessary for seed grinding.

Handyman ate seeds and other vegetation and used tools to scavenge predator kills. He was successful at this for more than half a million years. Finally, one group evolved into a larger variety that we call *Homo erectus*. They were about five feet six inches tall and had a braincase about the size of a modern four-year-old's.

Early Humans and Their Diet

Somewhere between 300,000 and 10,000 years ago, *Homo sapiens* arrived on the scene. They had the same subsistence diet as *Homo erectus* but had improved hunting methods. Plant food continued to predominate in their diet, but aquatic hunting and fishing techniques also appeared.

From about 10,000 years ago, the range of foodstuffs narrowed and cereals became much more prominent in the diet. Probably for the first time in human history, there were food surpluses, and the population thrived.

Dietary bulk and roughage were still very high in the diet. At the same time, malnutrition and starvation occurred, particularly affecting poorer populations.

This state of affairs continued until the 1800s when people began eating more. Now, refined carbohydrates assumed more importance, and the intake of salts and fats began increasing.

Even worse, all this food was being obtained with little physical exertion by those who were doing most of the eating. There were large city populations by now, and the city folk were lazily grazing off the efforts of the smaller population of farmers.

Obesity and colonic disorders began to increase among the populations of these developed countries, as did cardiovascular disorders linked to stress, salt intake, and high cholesterol levels.

The intake of surplus calories became common, and the average body size increased. Human milk as infant food was widely abandoned or rarely used—which proved to be one of our first major mistakes.

People stopped breastfeeding. It grew out of fashion, so to speak. As a result, we harmed our health even more. A species that developed for 4 million years on mother's milk was now getting most of its milk from cows. The result was the loss of such health-producing nutrients as colustrum—which can only be found in mother's milk—and is packed with vitamins and minerals.

Today's Food

In the last thirty years, things have gotten worse. Not only has the air we breathe gotten to be dangerous, but also the food we eat and the water we drink. I often tell my patients that the American diet of today is not fit for human consumption, because it's high in fat and cholesterol from meat—not to mention all the sugar we consume.

In addition, all kinds of pollutants are getting into our food. The additives alone that food manufacturers use are enough to kill us. We have also begun to introduce newly invented artificial compounds into our foods that have almost completely unknown consequences for the biochemistry of the liver.

These compounds may be affecting our brain, nervous system, hormone system, cardiovascular system, and even our immune system. And even though we have absolutely no idea what the long-term effects of these chemicals are, we still permit them to be put in our food, including baby food.

For quite some time, the refined foods of Western countries have been regarded as the best diet in the world. This view is now being challenged. Just look at the obesity problems we have in this country and the increase in diseases like diabetes.

High sugar intake and low physical activity have become characteristic of industrialized countries and are widely recognized as the causes of many health problems, including diabetes.

The refined carbohydrates we consume by the pounds in white flour and processed foods are also causing us health problems. Refining permits these carbohydrates to be quickly absorbed by the body, where, like sugar, they cause a sudden rise of glucose level in the blood. (Another danger of processed foods is that they usually contain hidden sugars.)

The body responds to this sudden rise of glucose with a strong secretion of insulin. This may not be a problem for highly active people, but for sedentary people, it's a disaster.

The hormone insulin directs unused glucose in the blood to be stored as fat tissue. And an excess of fat can lead to many health problems—including tooth and gum disease.

So, next time you treat yourself to sugar-rich food, processed foods or commercially baked goods, take a 10–20-minute run or brisk walk before your insulin lays down your extra glucose as new body fat! That brisk walk may help you to avoid many health problems.

Eating complex carbohydrates—meaning nonstarchy vegetables like asparagus and broccoli—does not cause a sudden rise of the glucose level in your blood, because your body absorbs these carbohydrates more slowly.

When you eat such alkalizing fruits and vegetables, the insulin secretion into the blood is also slower, although there is still a little extra insulin and glucose that enter your bloodstream to form new body fat.

When you think about our ancestors and the way we've evolved, it's surprising that we have survived as a species. But we won't survive if we do not wake up and take a close look at what we eat. We also need to change our rather sedentary lifestyles by exercising more.

Speaking of exercise, that doesn't mean having to weight-lift or anything that is very strenuous. As a matter of fact, the best exercises are easy and simple to do. One of the most effective ways to tone the body is by walking.

Our bodies are designed for walking. This is the way we, as a species, have gotten food for millions of years. Our primitive ancestors walked and walked and walked.

We evolved to walk, not to sit in front of a TV for hours every day watching soap operas or Judge Judy. We don't really need to do a lot of hard physical exercise—though that's a good way to keep fit—basically, we need to walk.

Walking still is the best overall exercise. We come from hunter-gatherers with the emphasis on "gatherers." This means that way back then, people spent a good portion of their day walking about and getting roots, vegetables, seeds, berries, etc., for food. So get moving if you want to stay healthy and have a better quality of life.

Run, Walk, Fast, Detoxify

So, here we are, driving our cars and going to fast-food restaurants to eat or buying poor quality convenience foods. As we get older, we get aches and pains, our blood pressure goes up, arthritis starts to set in, and the risk of heart attacks increases.

Nowadays, older people are also getting more and more tooth decay, which rarely happened previously. Tooth decay used to be primarily a childhood problem, because your body chemistry and mouth bacteria changed to protect against such decay as you aged.

Not anymore! There is not only a marked increase in tooth decay in older people, but in gum disease as well. Age is not to blame. The real cause is poor diet.

I'm 50 plus years old, and whenever I mention that to people, they usually act surprised. They often say that I look great for my age and that they thought I was about forty.

Well, it's not that I'm a Tom Cruise lookalike, but I am healthy and many people my age aren't. I also exercise fairly regularly and eat the proper foods. When I get up in the morning, and if the weather permits, I go out and run three to five miles. It's very quiet up in Woodstock, New York, where I live, and the early morning hours are magical. I use this time to meditate as well as to exercise.

I run, then walk for a while, and then run again. I devised this regimen because I feel it's close to what primitive men used to do—they ran and walked, ran and walked.

When I get home, I do some sit-ups followed by breakfast. It's usually some kind of fruit with various kinds of supplements. Lunch is another handful of supplements with a salad. For dinner, more vegetables and more supplements—usually phytonutrients which are made from whole foods.

Many people at midlife become ill from nutritional causes, whether they know it or not. They are not confined to bed, they still work, and some even exercise—but they're not healthy. They're just not eating the right foods. That's why they look older.

Fasting is also important. We know that the food supply of the hunter-gatherers that we evolved from must have run short from time to time and that they did not eat for a day or two. This is why a fast every now and then is actually good for you. It helps us to clean out our system.

Compared to early humans, we have another disadvantage. They knew how to recognize predators. If you were out foraging for food and you suddenly saw a saber-toothed tiger start to head your way, it didn't take much to realize you had to get out of there quickly.

Today's predators, however, are much more sophisticated, and unfortunately, they belong to our own species. They prey on us via advertising, getting us to spend money on useless foods and other products that can lead to poor health—and sometimes even kill us!

That's our second biggest mistake—listening to the manufacturers of poor-quality foods tell us that drinking Diet Coke is better than juicing organic fruits to refresh yourself. We're eating what the predators have convinced us to eat, instead of following our own instincts.

Liver-Gallbladder Flush

For overall cleansing, I recommend an occasional liver-gallbladder flush. Earlier, I mentioned that the color of the tongue is a factor in my oral diagnosis. A yellowish coating, for example, could indicate that my patient was developing problems in his or her liver or gallbladder.

If there are no medical problems that preclude treatment, a simple liver-gallbladder flush can be an effective method of starting my patient back on the road to health.

This flush is one you should try even if you are perfectly healthy—it has great value in preserving good health.

Many kinds of liver-gallbladder flushes are effective. My favorite flush consists of a three-day fast on olive oil and lemon juice, followed by six days on olive oil, lemon, and juices of carrot, spinach, beet, and cucumber. It's an old, old remedy.

Remember when you were a kid and had a cold or a flu? Your mother used to make you take a lot of juice. That's really what you were doing—cleansing your body.

Morning is the best time for flushing and cleansing the system. Start your day with the following:

Cold-pressed extra virgin olive oil, 2 tablespoons
Juice of one large or two small lemons
Juice of one or two grapefruit
Garlic cloves, one to four
Cayenne pepper, a dash

Place all the ingredients in a blender and blend until well mixed. After drinking the flush, follow with two cups of herbal tea or plain hot water. If you are concerned about smelling of garlic, you can use odorless garlic or take chlorophyll tablets to reduce the garlic odor.

You also might be interested in knowing that in her book *Healthy Healing*, author Linda Rector Page claims that enemas using garlic, coffee, or wheatgrass enhance the healing process.

Body-Cleansing Diet

As with a liver-gallbladder flush, most people can benefit from an occasional cleanse. Here is a pleasant diet that will help your body to rid itself of toxins. You should follow this diet for two weeks. For optimum health, I'd suggest that you do such a cleanse twice a year.

Midmorning
Eat a grapefruit or have a glass of fruit or vegetable juice.

Lunch
Fruit or vegetable salad. Do not mix. Use only fresh fruits or vegetables and cold-pressed oils, lemons, or other citrus fruits or herbs for dressings.

Midafternoon
Sprout snack (sprouts with tomatoes, onion, avocado, tamari sauce, olive oil, or lemons).

Dinner
Fruit or vegetable salad and/or baked or steamed vegetables. Try to keep this meal smaller than lunch.

After Dinner
Fruit or vegetable juice.

This cleansing process can be intensified by drinking at least ten glasses of liquid each day. While on a cleansing or detox diet, you may feel tired or like you have the flu or a bad cold.

This is part of the healing process and need not be a cause for alarm. After this kind of cleanse, it's important to introduce foods slowly. The following supplements should be taken during this detoxification period.

You'll notice that I suggest supplements such as L-carnitine, milk thistle, and liver extracts. All of these supplements are basically designed to help invigorate your liver.

Choline, 1 g per day
Omega-3 oil capsules, twice per day
L-carnitine, 500 mg, twice per day
L-methionine, 1 g per day
Milk thistle, 70–200 mg, three times per day
Liver extracts, 500 mg, three times per day
Selenium, 200 mcg per day

I hope, by now, that you see the value of proper diet for healthy teeth and a healthy body. By concentrating on proper nutrition, getting the right amount of exercise, reducing stress, and eliminating toxins from your body every once in a while through a fast or a flush, you will optimize your overall health.

CHAPTER 6

Tooth Decay and Toothaches: Getting to the Root of the Problem

What's in a Tooth?

Most dentists are happy if their patients pass a toothbrush over their teeth and floss once in a while. But if you want to prevent tooth decay, then you've got to focus on how you take care of those structures in your mouth.

A tooth is an organ adapted to tear and grind food. The visible tooth is simply an enamel coating that covers a softer tissue underneath called *dentin*. The middle of the tooth is a *pulp* cavity, and it contains nerve endings and blood vessels.

The enamel which covers the tooth is a crystalline form of calcium and is one of the body's hardest substances. The enamel protects the tooth from abrasive wear and tear.

In addition to breaking up food, teeth help us to say words and keep our facial muscles from caving in. Like other body organs, teeth have their own blood circulation and nerve supply.

Under the gum line, the dentin is covered with a substance called *cementum*, which is similar to bone. This cementum keeps the tooth attached to the gum and jawbone. A tooth is also held in the jawbone by collagen fibers that run from the tooth to the bone, with the bone forming a sheath around the tooth's membrane.

The gum tissue, derived from embryonic skin, covers the entire area and protects everything from infection. Normal gum tissue is wrapped tightly around the tooth, although there is a slight space, usually 2 to 3 millimeters deep, called a *pocket*.

The first tooth buds appear when a fetus is five weeks old. These buds undergo changes as cells multiply and tissue develops. When the buds harden into something resembling an adult tooth, it erupts from the gum.

Of the two sets of teeth a person has in a lifetime, the first—called baby teeth—erupt within the first year of life. The second set of teeth usually develops at about age six, starting with the molars and ending with the wisdom teeth between the ages of eighteen and twenty-one.

The second set of teeth pushes out the first set. There is no need for alarm when a child between five and seven has two sets of teeth. This is a passing stage due to the adult teeth coming in slightly behind the baby teeth, causing a shark-like appearance. This is normal and ends as soon as the adult teeth fully erupt.

Once your second and final set of teeth are in place, it's up to you and your dentist to keep your mouth a healthy place free of unwanted bacteria.

Tooth Decay

Let's get to the root of the problem right here. Despite what television commercials might try to tell us, brushing your teeth with Colgate or rinsing with Listerine may not prevent tooth decay.

We should not think of our teeth as small rock-like structures attached to the bones of the mouth. Think of them, instead, as being similar to coral reefs. If the marine environment is not in balance, these reefs, which are connected to each other, will die. Similarly, if the mouth environment is unbalanced, teeth will decay and possibly later die.

Such an imbalance comes about when the body's alkaline-acid ratios are upset and the mouth is too acidic. This acidity strips the tooth enamel of minerals, which weakens it and makes it more vulnerable to attack by bacteria, and ultimately to decay. This process is called *demineralization.*

Ordinarily, saliva bathes the mouth in an alkaline (nonacidic) solution that neutralizes all the acidity and actually remineralizes the teeth. The saliva also washes away leftover bits of food, and helps with the digestion process.

But when your saliva turns acidic because of too many sweets, fats, dairy, and other foodstuffs, bacteria are not kept in check and they begin to feed on food remnants in the teeth.

These nasty bacteria, along with carbohydrate waste, stick to the teeth and tongue and hold the acid close to the tooth where it eats away at the enamel. This is the beginning of tooth decay.

OH, MY ACHING TOOTH!

Many dental problems affecting the teeth result from the following:

- Not getting the proper nutrients in your diet, causing an acidic environment in the mouth.
- Not properly absorbing nutrients. Patients with dental and other health problems sometimes bring to my office a long list of the nutrients that they are taking. When people take a lot of supplements and are still not absorbing nutrients, I usually suggest they go for a medical checkup.
- Excessive stress. This can cause a depletion of the body's minerals at a surprisingly rapid rate.
- Hormonal imbalances. If the imbalance is due to an illness, some glands may not be functioning properly, and mineral deficiencies can be the result.

Anthropologist Morris Steggerda once did an interesting study with the Maya Indians in Mexico's Yucatan Peninsula. He discovered that when these Indians ate their traditional diet of corn, beans, vegetables, and fruit, little tooth decay occurred. Those who ate a more modern diet—including sweets—very quickly developed toothaches.

Although we will be discussing the dangers of sugar in Chapter 11, I'd like to mention here that the average American eats 130 pounds of sugar a year, which is about a half cup of sugar a day.

The soft drink industry, meanwhile, reports that the average soft drink consumption per person is close to 500 bottles a year, or 1.5 bottles a day. That can feed a lot of harmful oral bacteria.

To help avoid demineralization of your teeth, I suggest you follow the recommendations in this book to eat more fruits and vegetables and limit the amount of sugar and animal protein in your diet.

I'd also suggest that, in addition to brushing after each meal, you take multivitamin and multimineral supplements during or after your meals—especially if you are too rushed or otherwise distracted to eat properly.

The following vitamins are excellent for overall good health, but you don't need to take them all at once. You can even take your vitamin supplements one day, and your mineral supplements the next. (For more information on vitamins, see Chapter 9. Learn more about minerals in Chapter 10.)

HIGH-PRIORITY SUPPLEMENTS

Vitamins

Vitamin A and beta-carotene complex, 5,000–50,000 IU
Vitamin B-complex, 200–250 mg
Vitamin C, entire complex, 1,000 mg
Vitamin D, 400–800 IU
Vitamin E, 400–1,200 IU
Vitamin K, 100 mcg

Minerals

Boron, 3 mg
Calcium, 1,000 mg
Chromium, 200 mcg
Copper, 2 mg
Iodine, 150 mcg

Iron, 15 mg
Magnesium, 500 mg
Manganese, 15 mg
Selenium, 50 mg
Zinc, 22 mg

Other Important Supplements
Choline, 350 mg
Coenzyme Q10, 100 mg
EPA, 250 mg
Folic acid, 400 mcg
Garlic, 250 mg
GLA, 100 mg
Glutathione, 500 mg
Inositol, 100–500 mg
L-carnitine, 1,000–5,000 mg
PABA, 50–100 mg

Herbs to Reduce Tooth Decay

In addition to a proper diet and vitamin supplementation, herbal preparations can also be helpful in keeping your teeth and gums healthy. I've been using herbs to help my patients overcome a variety of oral problems since 1978, and have even developed a mouthwash and toothpaste chock full of herbs which you can find in most drug stores. (See the Resource Guide at the back of this book.)

At the end of this book, you will find a chapter containing many herbs that are healthy for the gums and teeth. These are a few of them that I am particularly fond of in my never-ending battle against tooth decay and gum disease. NOTE: Because each of these herbs is unique, be sure to consult the preparation instructions on the package.

• **Dandelion.** Excellent for adding minerals to teeth. Place the herb in boiling water for 15 to 20 minutes then let stand overnight. You can drink this tea or use it as a rinse. This herb can also be purchased in powdered form and mixed with water to form a thick paste. Apply this paste to the teeth and leave for a few minutes. Repeat this every few hours.

• **Licorice.** Can reduce tooth decay because of its antibacterial properties. Licorice root powder mixed with water and applied to the affected area is highly effective.

• **Alfalfa, Dandelion, Horsetail.** A combination of these herbs can help to strengthen the tooth's enamel and reduce sensitivity. They are also a natural source of fluoride, which helps to fight tooth decay. A high-mineral drink can be made from these herbs. You can also drink it as a tea or use as a rinse.

Always remember that a decaying tooth will continue to deteriorate until the tooth is completely destroyed. While all the above supplements and herbs are helpful, seeking professional care is even more important.

If you have good oral hygiene but are experiencing tooth decay problems, it's time for you and a professional to take a good look at the type of substances that are going into your body and causing these infections.

Keep in mind that if infections are debilitating your teeth, what are they doing to other parts of your body?

STUNTED GROWTH AND BABIES' TEETH

Researchers believe that tooth decay in early childhood can interfere with physical growth. Growth patterns are changed not because of tooth decay, but because of the mineral imbalances that caused the tooth decay in the first place.

This is because a thin layer of fluids and food will stay on an infant's teeth. This layer contains sugars which will promote bacterial growth and, in the case of juices, acids that will weaken the tooth structure.

If your child's teeth are in a decayed state and broken down, that child is going to tend to eat soft and squishy foods. Instead of munching on carrots, he or she will most likely favor something like a Twinkie or a slice of pizza.

The youngster won't get vital, growth-promoting vitamins and minerals eating these kinds of foods, and will grow at a slower pace than children with healthy teeth.

When the decayed teeth are treated, the child's eating patterns are likely to return to normal, and growth resumes.

Dentists and doctors also warn against letting babies between the ages of four to six months old—or whenever their first teeth come in—fall asleep while sucking on bottles containing milk, juice, or sweet liquids. They also suggest wiping a baby's gums with a damp cloth after feeding. This will prevent a thin layer of food or fluid from remaining on the infant's teeth. This layer contains sugars that can promote bacterial growth. In the case of juices, these can contain acids that will weaken the tooth's structure.

Toothaches

Tooth pain can be one of the worst agonies you will ever experience. Your body is telling you that something is wrong and needs your attention right now. A toothache usually occurs when the tooth nerve is damaged or dying.

A dull, throbbing pain is likely to be caused by an infected nerve, while a sharp, stabbing pain or a pain that occurs whenever you eat is more likely to be the result of tooth decay. Wisdom teeth coming in, inflamed gums, and excessive grinding of teeth can also cause toothaches.

Whatever your problem, your tooth is desperately signaling you, and expecting some emergency first aid. The best thing to do, of course, is see your dentist immediately.

Even if the pain suddenly stops, do not cancel that dental appointment! An absence of pain simply means that the symptom is temporarily suppressed. It doesn't mean that the cause of the problem has gone away.

If you can't immediately get an appointment with your dentist, here are some helpful tips that can help ease your discomfort until you do:

- Stay away from extreme temperatures. Don't eat very hot or cold foods.

- Don't eat hard foods. Sometimes a toothache can be caused by a hairline fracture.

Toothache-Fighting Herbs

The following herbs may help give you temporary relief from a toothache until you see your dentist:

• **Clove Oil.** One of the most effective natural pain relievers. Because clove oil is strong and can irritate sensitive gums, dilute it with an equal amount of olive or vegetable oil.

Place some on a small piece of cotton and gently apply this to the affected area. The relief should be rapid and last for up to an hour. Whole cloves are also effective, but the oil is more penetrating.

• **Garlic, Myrrh.** These herbs can also be applied locally for pain relief. Whole garlic can be crushed and rubbed onto the teeth. However, if you plan on having any sort of social life, it is better to purchase tinctures of garlic and myrrh from your health food store. Combine the two tinctures. I have found them more useful this way than used separately.

• **Calendula, Chamomile, Echinacea, Tumeric, Bee Propolis.** Calendula and chamomile soothe and help to heal tissues, while echinacea and turmeric fight infections.

Mix these powdered herbs with a little water and bee propolis until you have a muddy solution. Apply this directly to the infected area. Keep the application on the tooth for as long as you like.

• **Plantain.** Try plantain (either root or leaves) powder mixed with water. Apply directly to the tooth.

• **Cinquefoil.** In addition to helping with tooth pain, it is also very helpful for gum disease. This is another one of my favorites, and can be found in most health food stores. Use as with plantain.

• **Licorice.** Mix with water and apply to the area of pain. Very effective. A tea made out of licorice is also quite effective.

• **Ginger, Slippery Elm.** Helps to rapidly reduce pain. A tincture (in liquid form) or powder can both be used.

• **Gypsum, Pulsatilla, Long Pepper, Prickly Ash.** Prickly ash comes in powder form. The others are available in tinctures. Apply to the affected area.

• **Balm.** Make balm into a tea and use it as a rinse in the area where you are experiencing pain.

• **German Chamomile.** You may be able to purchase this at your health food store as a tincture. If not, go to a herbalist and get two dried flowers. Add them to a half cup of boiling water. Let it cool and take a mouthful at the time. Slosh it around the affected area.

• **Mullein.** This herb seems to augment the properties of other pain relievers. Use it as a tincture with balm or German chamomile.

• **Rose.** Good for toothaches. Boil the petals of red roses for five minutes and then steep for another ten. Mix with a small amount of any type of wine and rinse.

• **Cinnamon, Fenugreek, Sesame.** Try a rinse of two parts cinnamon to one part fenugreek and one part sesame seed (black seeds are the best) along with half a cup of water. Boil for five minutes and then steep for another five.

• **Pennyroyal.** Works well as a tea to help remove tooth pain.

• **White Willow, Rosemary, Wood Betty, Heartsease, Skullcap, Valerian, Red Raspberry, Ginger.** Try a combination of these herbs. Take equal amounts of each and make a tea.

• **Echinacea, Goldenseal, Cayenne Pepper, Myrrh, Yarrow, Marshmallow, Black Walnut, Turmeric.** This potent combination may jump-start the healing process. Take equal amounts of each and make a tea.

• **White Oak, Goldenseal.** These herbs will help to reduce pain and swelling. Use as a rinse.

Saliva: Nature's Antibacterial

Saliva is extremely important to your oral good health. In addition to helping digest food and remove leftover food particles, saliva carries minerals to the teeth. It also has antibacterial properties.

People whose salivary glands are dysfunctional and don't secrete sufficient saliva are apt to suffer from attacks of oral bacteria, viruses, and fungi. Even rinsing your mouth with water after eating helps neutralize decay, and can cut your bad bacteria levels by a third.

If a pharmaceutical company manufactured saliva, it could market it as a wonder drug! This is because proteins in saliva can:

- Kill bacteria.
- Stop bacteria from sticking to teeth, thereby preventing them from starting an infection.
- Cause bacteria to clump together for easier disposal.
- Neutralize bacterial toxins.

What causes a depleted saliva flow? The likeliest culprits are prescription or over-the-counter drugs. More than four hundred drugs reduce the secretion of saliva, including some decongestants, antihistamines, antihypertensives, and antidepressants.

A dry mouth can also be caused by anxiety, radiation therapy, and the autoimmune disorder known as Sjogren's Syndrome. Holistic physician and best-selling author Andrew Weil says that if you suspect a medication is causing dry mouth, ask your doctor or pharmacist to change your medication.

If changing your medication doesn't yield any improvement, Dr. Weil suggests the following natural do's and don'ts.

Do	Don't
Sip water often.	Drink alcohol.
Add lemon juice to drinking water.	Use alcohol-containing mouthwashes.
Suck sugar-free lozenges.	Eat salty food.
Chew sugar-free gum.	Drink coffee or caffeinated beverages.
Massage the underside of your jawbones.	Smoke.

CHILDREN'S CAVITIES: LEAD VS. VITAMIN C

According to researchers at the University of Rochester and the Children's Hospital Medical Center of Cincinnati, high levels of lead in the body may account for 11 percent of the cavities in children's teeth.

Studies done at these hospitals also showed that children with high levels of vitamin C had lower levels of lead. Ever since lead was removed from household paint and gasoline nationwide, far fewer children show dangerous levels of this metal in their bloodstreams.

However, the danger still exists. The Centers for Disease Control and Prevention claim that nearly a million children in the United States presently have unhealthy levels of lead in their bodies, which can have more serious consequences than tooth decay. Brain damage is one of them.

If you want to make certain that your child does not develop tooth decay due to high levels of lead, make sure that he or she gets plenty of vitamin C—and it wouldn't hurt if you got plenty of it, too.

Because the amount of vitamin C for children depends on weight and age, check with your doctor for the appropriate dosage.

CHAPTER 7

Saving Your Gums

Here's a startling statistic to sink your teeth into. More teeth are lost due to gum disease than to tooth decay. In fact, 75 percent of American adults over the age of thirty-five suffer from some form of periodontal disease, according to the American Dental Association.

Periodontal disease takes two forms: simple gum inflammation called *gingivitis*, which is caused by bacteria, and a more severe gum infection called *periodontitis*, which may lead to tooth loss.

Gingivitis results from plaque and tartar that irritate the gum or periodontal tissue. Regular brushing and flossing can often prevent this condition from developing. The more advanced state of gum disease—periodontitis—occurs when inflammation of the gums is accompanied by bone and ligament destruction.

A strong immune system, healthy gums and bones, and bacterial control all help prevent periodontitis. Regular dental visits are a must, as is dedicated oral hygiene such as brushing after meals, cleaning between the teeth using floss, using a water irrigator to stimulate the gums, and even scrubbing the tongue with a brush or a tongue scraper before you go to sleep.

If your gums aren't bleeding when you brush, or are not inflamed or receding, that doesn't necessarily mean you do not have gum disease. Periodontitis often shows no symptoms, and only a checkup will reveal if this disease is present or not. So avoid problems and check with your dentist every three or four months.

GUM DISEASE MAY BE INHERITED

A study in the *Journal of Medical Genetics* indicates that the health of your gums is not just determined by what you eat and how well you brush your teeth, but by your genes as well. In fact, genes may play as important a role as diet and dental hygiene in the development of gum disease. An international team of researchers discovered that changes in a gene for the enzyme Cathepsin C are responsible for a condition known as Papillon-Lefvre syndrome. Symptoms include scaly, warty thickening of the skin and erosion of the soft tissues lining the mouth and connecting bones along with inflammation of the gums. Cathepsin C, found in skin and bone cells, activates several of the chemicals controlling immune and inflammatory responses. The scientists have found that different mutations of the gene are responsible for two other syndromes: Haim-Munk syndrome, in which the mouth tissues are not so badly affected, but in which the skin symptoms are more severe and extensive, and prepubertal periodontitis, a rare but rapidly progressive gum disease, but with no skin symptoms, that affects young children.

A healthy immune system is most important in battling this disease. Low resistance provides a prime environment for harmful bacteria to multiply to dangerous proportions.

Just as a mouth that becomes too acidic can cause cavities, so can it result in gum disease. One of the primary causes of periodontal disease, however, is excessive stress.

While a certain amount of stress is considered normal, excessive stress can take its toll on the teeth and body. Stress has not only been linked to periodontal problems, but can also interfere with digestion, alter brain chemistry, and even increase the heart rate.

How many of you reading this book took final exams while in college and had bleeding gums during that stressful period? I'd bet one out of three of my readers answer "yes" to that question.

This happens all the time when college students have finals and are under extra stress. At that time of the year my office is inundated with calls from students who are suffering great pain from their bleeding gums. I give them some natural remedies, throw in a cleaning, and when their finals end, the condition disappears.

I remember one particular patient—her name was Mary—who arrived in my office on a spring afternoon. Mary was a twenty-seven-year-old accounting major. Her gums were bleeding and she was in a lot of pain. I said, "Mary, what's going on?"

"My diet's good, everything in my life is good," she replied.

I looked steadily at her for a few moments. "Well, if it's so good, why are you here?"

"I don't know, but you've got to help me get rid of this condition," she pleaded.

After talking to her, I learned that Mary's diet was, indeed, good, that she exercised regularly, and was in a good relationship. Then all of a sudden it hit me. It was June.

"Mary, are you taking finals now?" I asked her.

She nodded. "Yes, and they're killing me."

I laughed. I said, "This will go away as soon as you're through with your finals." I put her on a herbal mouth rinse, and two days later when her finals were finished, she was fine.

If you have gum problems, it could also mean that you are suffering from an acid/alkaline imbalance. That's why diet and eating the proper foods are so important for good oral health. (See Chapter 8: Good Foods, Bad Foods.)

Let's take a closer look at the anatomy of periodontal or gum disease. To begin with, you need to understand how teeth are held in the mouth. They are not directly embedded into the jawbones, but are surrounded by tissue called the *periodontal membrane*.

This tissue, among other things, acts as a shock absorber for the teeth. The periodontal membrane is actually a continuation of the gum tissue that covers all the bone and tooth parts in the mouth, except for the tooth crown (the part we see).

The periodontal membrane has thousands of tiny fibers, called *pe-*

riodontal ligaments, that go from the membrane and attach to the teeth and bone. In a normal, healthy mouth, there is always a slight space between tooth and bone called a *pocket*, which is usually 1 to 2 millimeters (about an eighth of an inch) deep.

This all changes when peridontal disease strikes.

Periodontal disease is basically caused by bacteria. Poor oral hygiene allows plaque to form on the teeth. These deposits permit the growth of bacteria that cause inflammation of the gums.

The bacteria also release minute amounts of toxins that break down the gum tissue, thereby helping the infection to progress. Plaque is an invisible sticky film of saliva and food residue that constantly forms on the teeth.

Bacteria help to create plaque and they thrive within it. Unless removed, plaque formed along the gumline can lead to gum disease. When left untreated, plaque at or below the gumline hardens into tartar.

While flossing and brushing can remove plaque, the removal of rocklike tartar requires the use of dental instruments.

As the infection progresses, the gum tissue becomes red, instead of its normal healthy pink color. The tissue also gets puffy. Bleeding occurs, especially when you floss or brush. Bacteria then migrate into the pocket and begin to destroy the periodontal membrane.

The toxins produced by the bacteria also destroy the bone in the immediate area. The normal, healthy pocket can be deepened from 1–2 to 3–4 millimeters, and in severe cases to 7–10 millimeters or more.

Over time, after the supporting periodontal ligaments have been completely destroyed, the teeth involved become loosened and eventually fall out. Inflammation of the gums, known as gingivitis, is often the first symptom we have that this is going on.

Aside from bacteria, periodontal disease can result from mechanical problems, usually from excessive pressure on a tooth, which can be the result of a teeth-grinding habit or of an uneven bite. Dental restorations that do not fit properly can also cause the gum tissue around the restoration to become irritated.

Most traditional dentists will tell you that bacterial infection causes tooth decay and gum disease. Insofar as it goes, this explanation is correct. But it doesn't go far enough.

What these dentists don't tell you is that the infection may have been caused because the patient's body chemistry was out of balance in the first place, leading to a weakened immune system and less resistance to harmful bacteria.

So what do they do? These conventional dentists focus all their efforts on removing the symptoms rather than trying to get to the cause of the problem. What this means is that before long you'll be right back in that dental seat.

EIGHT WARNING SIGNS OF GUM DISEASE

- Brushing causes gums to bleed.
- Persistent bad breath.
- Soft, swollen, or tender gums.
- Pus appears when you put pressure on gums or teeth.
- Loose teeth.
- Receding gums.
- Your bite changes because of teeth shifting.
- Denture fit changes.

Stop Tartar Before It Begins

The best way to prevent tartar is to stop the buildup of plaque on your teeth. You can rid your teeth of newly formed plaque by thorough daily dental care.

Brush first with a dry soft-bristle toothbrush. Use gentle side-to-side strokes in which the brush is half on the gums and half on the teeth. Gum disease usually starts beneath the gums, so clean under the gumline and between teeth with unwaxed dental floss—although I have nothing against the waxed kind either.

Rubber tip stimulators, which are available at most drug stores, and wooden dental sticks should be used after you brush and floss. Lastly, brush your teeth and tongue with a good herbal toothpaste available in most health food stores and even drug stores.

We all know that for urinary infections, cranberry juice can often stop those infections dead in their tracks. What you might not be aware of is that cranberry juice also helps to fight plaque because it also seems to interfere with bacteria forming plaque on teeth.

Erwin I. Weiss, a researcher at Tel Aviv University, tested cranberry juice extract on decay-causing oral bacteria along with other substances. The antioxidant found in cranberries, polyphenol, seemed to be the ingredient that best prevented the bacteria from forming plaque.

But don't go running out to your nearest grocery store to purchase a jug of cranberry juice. According to the Israeli researcher, "the commercially available cranberry juice cocktail is not suitable for oral hygiene purposes. The product is sweetened with up to 12 percent fructose and dextrose, which may promote plaque accumulation and tooth decay."

Instead, buy unsweetened cranberry juice at your local health food store and dilute it to taste.

Conventional Treatment of Periodontal Disease

Most mainstream dentists recognize two main methods of treating gum disease: surgical removal of the diseased tissue and low dosages of antibiotics.

While both methods have good success rates, a large number of patients return with the same problem a few years later. Personally, I don't think that reinforces the idea that dentists are healers.

During surgery, the gums are cut and peeled back to reveal the tooth's roots. Infected tissue and tartar are removed. The roots may then be scraped. Sometimes bone is grafted. Then the gums are sewn back up. After the gums have healed, the teeth may be extremely sensitive to temperature, certain foods, or brushing.

Antibiotics usually consist of a small dose of tetracycline, injected in the infected area. This kills the local germs and the infection disappears. One problem with this method, however, is that your body can build up resistance to the antibiotic. Such resistance is already happening on a wide scale with drugs designed to combat tuberculosis.

In fact, we are now seeing "super bugs" that are not affected by normal antibiotics and that, in some instances, actually thrive on the drugs that are supposed to eradicate them!

Holistic Treatment of Periodontal Disease

Holistic dentists are trying to develop new ways to more effectively combat periodontal disease. They prefer to try and control this disease through oral hygiene, a good diet rich in nutrients and high in fiber, supplementation with vitamins and minerals, and avoidance of harmful substances such as cigarettes and coffee.

These methods don't merely attack the symptoms, but initiate a change in the body's chemistry and enhance the immune system. This whole-body approach has proven to be not only quite effective, but also safer and less expensive than conventional treatments.

Dentistry has made many wonderful technological advances over the past decade, and will continue to do so. I strongly believe it is now time to combine this technology with alternative healing modalities.

My philosophy has always been: keep it simple. The least invasive technique should always be tried first. I never consider surgery as an option during the first six months of treatment for gum disease. And over the years, I have successfully treated even advanced cases of periodontal disease nonsurgically.

One such success story involves one of my patients, whom I will call Roger. At fifty-four, Roger seemed to be in reasonable health. Yet he noticed that he was beginning to develop gum problems.

Five years earlier he had undergone periodontal surgery, and swore that he'd never do it again. One day he heard me speak on a local radio show, and called for an appointment.

My examination showed that Roger had bleeding gums with generalized bone loss and areas of infection around some of his teeth. I had him do a diet analysis. Roger was in a very stressful work situation and he had no time for or interest in proper nutrition. His body chemistry was seriously out of balance.

I placed him on supplements, including vitamins C and E, calcium, minerals, and phytonutrients, which are live plant extracts.

Then he went on my fast-alkalizing diet, which I will describe in the next chapter. I also cleaned the pockets between his teeth and gums, and gave him instructions on how to use herbal rinses, which I will also talk about later on.

Four months later Roger was back in my office. His gum tissue was now healthy and the bone loss seemed to have stopped. He was feeling better and told me he was staying on the diet, calling it "a lifestyle change."

My Periodontal Protocol

First Visit

- A discussion of your general health, followed by temporomandibular joint testing (see page 11) and a thorough oral examination.
- Discussion of gum problems encountered, their causes, and healing options.
- Recommended diet.
- Recommended supplements.

Second Visit

- Review of gum problems, diet, and supplements.
- Most effective use of dental floss and toothbrush.
- Most effective use of irrigator.

Third and Fourth Visits

- Deep cleansing of teeth: cleansing of pockets between teeth and gums, scaling of teeth, root planing, and tooth polishing.

Fifth Visit

- This visit is necessary only when work remains to be done or if complications occur.

Supplements for Gum Disease

I prefer getting my vitamins and minerals from whole foods rather than supplements, because whole foods contain many factors not found in commercially produced multivitamins.

But in situations where your diet has been poor, or you are trying to reverse gum disease naturally, the following supplements may help you do so.

- Vitamin C, 2–4 g per day (taken as 500 mg every few hours)
- Calcium, 800 mg (take in a formula that comes with magnesium)
- Vitamin E, 200–400 IU per day
- Zinc picolinate, 30 mg per day
- Magnesium, 600 mg per day
- Beta-carotene complex, 2500 IU per day
- Coenzyme Q10, 100 mg per day
- Vitamin B complex, 15–25 mg per day
- Multivitamin/mineral, one per day

A colleague of mine, Dr. Richard Fischer, recommends daily servings of foods rich in vitamin C, such as broccoli, citrus fruits, peppers, and tomatoes, because decreased levels of vitamin C allow greater passage of harmful bacteria into the surrounding teeth.

I agree with this, and would also add some organic vitamin C supplements with bioflavonoids to this diet.

GUM DISEASE FIGHTERS

All of the following nutrients have been found effective in combating gum disease.

- Chlorella, 1 capsule per day
- Cilantro (Chinese parsley)
- Flaxseed oil, up to 2 tablespoons per day
- Garlic extract, 1200–2400 mg in two divided doses per day
- Glutathione, 150 mg in three divided doses per day

- Methionine, 600–1500 mg in three divided doses per day
- Grapeseed, 100 mg per day
- Parsley
- Probiotics

Ten Ways to Prevent Gum Disease

You've been exposed in this chapter to much new information about how to prevent or reverse periodontal disease. Let me try to sum up what I consider are the most important steps you can take in your war against gum disease:

- Pay close attention to your diet. Stay away from sugars and fats.
- Take vitamins, minerals, and herbs to boost your immune system.
- Maintain a conscientious oral hygiene program that includes brushing your teeth at least twice a day with a soft toothbrush.
- Visit your dentist regularly—every three or four months. Early degenerative diseases can be corrected.
- Eat more high-fiber foods such as fruits and vegetables.
- Massage your gums with your fingers when you get a chance.
- Go on a cleansing diet to eliminate toxins from your body.
- Avoid stress. It encourages the growth of harmful bacteria.
- Take calcium and vitamin C to promote good gum health.
- Become an educated consumer. Read up on homeopathic remedies, aromatherapy, Bach flower remedies, and other natural substances that promote healing.

Remember, nowhere does proper self-care pay off more than in the mouth. If you follow the recommendations in this chapter and elsewhere in the book, I promise you a better chance of keeping your teeth intact for the rest of your life.

CHAPTER 8

Good Foods, Bad Foods

I've long believed that by changing people's diets, I can bring about a positive change in both their dental and total physical health. Teeth start to decay when a person's diet is too acidic. They've been eating too much meat, dairy products, and sugar which, in turn, can cause saliva to become acidic.

As you know by now, when the saliva changes to such an acidic state, harmful bacteria have a field day. This doesn't happen when the mouth has a more alkaline environment.

Fruits and vegetables such as blueberries and broccoli, along with nuts, seeds, and certain proteins, are excellent alkalizing foods. They help the body assimilate bacteria-fighting vitamins, phytonutrients, and minerals.

The following list of foods will help you get the proper nutrition for the mouth and what ails it. You might notice citrus fruit on the list. Despite its acidity, citrus fruit helps reduce cavities by stimulating saliva.

Increase Intake of Alkalizing Foods

Alkalizing Fruits

Apple
Apricot
Avocado
Banana
Blackberry
Blueberry
Cherry
Citrus fruit
Currant, black and red
Date
Fig
Grape
Melon
Nectarine
Peach
Pear
Pineapple
Raspberry
Strawberry

Alkalizing Vegetables

Asparagus
Beets
Broccoli
Brussels sprouts
Cabbage
Carrot
Cauliflower
Celery
Chard
Collard greens
Cucumber
Eggplant

Kale
Kohlrabi
Lettuce
Mushrooms
Mustard greens
Onions
Parsnips
Peppers
Pumpkin
Rutabaga
Sea vegetables
Sprouts (all kinds)
Squashes
Tomato

Alkalizing Seasonings

Apple cider vinegar
Chili peppers
Cinnamon
Curry
Garlic
Ginger
Herbs (all)
Mustard
Salt

Alkalizing Sweetener

Stevia

Alkalizing Nuts and Seeds

Almond
Chestnut
Flaxseed
Millet
Pumpkin seed
Squash seed

Alkalizing Protein

Egg
Chicken breast
Cottage cheese, fat-free
Tofu
Whey protein powder
Yogurt

Alkalizing Beverages

Fruit juice, fresh and unsweetened
Herbal tea
Tea
Vegetable juice
Water

Decrease Intake of Acidifying Foods

Acidifying Vegetables

Black bean
Chickpea
Kidney bean
Lentil
Lima bean
Pinto bean
Potato
Red bean
Soybean
White bean

Acidifying Grains

Amaranth
Barley
Buckwheat
Corn

Oats
Quinoa
Rice
Rye
Wheat

Acidifying Dairy Products

Butter
Cheese
Milk

Acidifying Fats and Oils

Animal fats, all
Vegetable oils, all

Acidifying Sweeteners

Aspartame
Honey
Maple syrup
Molasses
Saccharin
Sugar

Acidifying Nuts

Brazil nut
Cashew
Filbert
Peanut
Pecan
Walnut

Acidifying Protein

Beef
Duck
Fish

Lamb
Lobster
Pork
Shellfish
Shrimp
Turkey

Acidifying Beverages

Beer
Soft drinks
Spirits
Wine

While individual requirements differ, a healthy person should probably aim for a mix of 80 percent alkalizing foods and 20 percent acidifying foods. The formula goes as follows:

80% Alkalizing Foods + 20% Acidifying Foods =
100% Slightly Alkaline Body Fluids

A mixed diet is best. Eating only alkalizing foods is not recommended for long-term good health. However, eating alkalizing foods almost exclusively for a relatively short time can de-acidify your body fluids.

Later on in this chapter, I will give you a fast-acting diet that will permit your body fluids to quickly make the change from an acidifying condition to one that is more alkaline.

YOUR FOOD DIARY

Before you take any steps to change your diet, you first need to take a hard look at what you actually eat every day. This involves writing down what you eat, the time you eat, and the amount.

For example, it's not sufficient to write in your chart: "Eggs and toast for breakfast." Were there three eggs fried in butter? Was the toast heavily covered with sugar-laden jam? How many cups of coffee? No juice? No vitamins?

Most smokers, when they start to keep an honest count, are surprised by the number of cigarettes they smoke each day. Nearly all of us, when we start to keep an accurate accounting of our food intake, are amazed at the amount we eat each day.

But it's not only the food quantity that is likely to surprise. The low quality of most of what we eat is often something we may have failed to notice before. You need accurate information before you can make meaningful changes in your diet.

When you keep a written record:

1. You become aware of the kind of food you eat.
2. You see the quantity you eat.
3. You see the quality of what you eat.

Too Much Protein

When we don't eat enough fruits and vegetables, and consume too much protein, animal fats, sugar-rich processed foods, and refined grains, we acidify our body fluids.

Excess protein in your diet can result in the following problems:

- Acidifies the body chemistry because of its abundant sulfur and phosphorus. These minerals change into sulfuric and phosphoric acids, thus depleting the body of necessary minerals.
- Impairs protein synthesis inside the cells.
- Lowers white blood cell production, which weakens the immune system.

Most Americans eat 80 to 120 grams of protein per day. The RDI is 63 grams of protein for adult males, and 50 grams for adult females. I believe that these numbers should be much lower.

In fact, for most people, 20 to 30 grams of protein in food should be sufficient. The following chart will give you an idea of the amount of protein in the foods you eat:

Food	Protein, grams
Steak, 8 oz.	64
Chicken, broiled, 4 oz.	33
Flounder, broiled, 4 oz.	27
Hamburger	25
Beef burrito	25
Almonds, 4 oz.	20
Milk, 1 cup	8
Beans, boiled, 2 cups	6–7
Egg	6

Too Many Animal Fats

We're talking about excess "bad" fats here—mostly animal fats. The average American diet seems to be sorely lacking in "good fats," such as Omega-3 and -6 fatty acids. The more good fats we have in our diet, the less we crave bad fats.

Excess animal fats are acidifying because they block oxygen from reaching cells, which slows down the cell's sodium-potassium pump and permits acidic waste products to accumulate within the cell. Acetic acid is also a by-product of fat metabolism, further acidifying the body.

Good Fats

Healthful omega fatty acids are essential in our diet. Because our bodies can't produce them, they must be obtained from outside sources.

The essential fatty acids play a major part in the manufacture of prostaglandins, hormonelike substances that are used by every cell in the body.

Prostaglandins regulate all of our body functions. In addition, they are used as structural parts of the cell membranes and help protect the cells from bacteria, toxins, carcinogens, viruses, allergens, and other factors intent on doing you harm.

SOURCES OF OMEGA FATTY ACIDS	
Omega-3	**Omega-6**
Salmon, sardines	Safflower oil
Flaxseeds, flaxseed oil	Sesame seeds
Green leafy vegetables	Soybeans
Soybeans	Sunflower seeds
Walnuts	Evening primrose oil

Omega-3 fatty acids are far more likely to be deficient in your diet than Omega-6. Flaxseeds are the richest alkalizing plant source for Omega-3.

Soybeans contain both Omega-3 and -6. If you don't like the taste of soy, chocolate, strawberry, or vanilla-flavored soy milk might be easier on your taste buds. You can find soy milk in cartons next to regular milk in many supermarkets.

Too Many Simple Carbohydrates

Sugar of all kinds, processed foods, and refined grains are simple carbohydrates. They are often lacking in minerals. To be metabolized, these carbohydrates must steal minerals from the body's reserves.

For example, eating sugar increases the excretion of calcium. These mineral losses are best restored by eating fruits and vegetables (complex carbohydrates). Nutrients in pill or capsule form also work, but whole foods deliver a wide spectrum of substances not found in artificial supplements.

TEN TOP FOODS FOR DENTAL HEALTH

Asparagus
Beets
Broccoli
Carrots
Celery
Cauliflower
Lettuce
Kale
Onions
Spinach

The Natural Dentist's Fast-Alkalizing Diet

How do you know how acid or alkaline your body fluids are? It's easy! Using widely available special litmus paper that changes color, you can actually check the alkalinity/acidity of your saliva and urine. We'll get to that in a few moments.

If after measuring your saliva and urine you see that your body fluids are too acid, you need to switch things around in your body. The following special diet that I have formulated will enable your body fluids to become more alkaline in a relatively short time. But as with all nutritional remedies, you need to give this diet time to work.

Some individuals may see improvements in less than a week. Others may require two or three weeks. If you have medical problems, you should check with a physician before going on this diet to see whether any modifications are needed.

Don't worry if you can't strictly adhere to this diet. Just try your best. The more you're able to follow it, the better you will feel. As the state of your health improves, following this diet will no longer be a chore but rather a tool for vital living.

Don't, however, stay on this diet for more than a month. After that, begin adding other foods, using this diet as a general guideline. By the way, you will notice that some of the foods in the diet are acidifying rather than alkalinizing. That's because, as I mentioned before, a strictly alkaline diet—except for a short amount of time when you are trying to change your body chemistry—is not good for you, either. To stay healthy you'll need to eat a variety of foods.

Alkaline Diet Menu

Breakfast

Fruit—any kind.

Lunch

Monday, Wednesday, Friday
> One or two kinds of fresh fruit in season (see "Alkalizing Fruits" list above)
> *or* apricots
> *or* figs, currants (dried fruit may be soaked)
> *and* avocado

Tuesday, Thursday, Saturday, Sunday
> Small *raw* vegetable salad (must have romaine lettuce and sprouts, plus two or three other vegetables)
> *and* avocado or rice cakes or 3 ounces of raw nuts (almonds, filberts, walnuts, pecans)

Dinner

Monday
> Large *raw* vegetable salad and baked potato or lentils or chickpeas
> *and,* if needed, one steamed vegetable (see "Alkalizing Vegetables" list above)

Tuesday
Large *raw* vegetable salad and baked yam or avocado.

Wednesday
Large *raw* vegetable salad and baked potato or corn or lentils *and*, if needed, one steamed vegetable.

Thursday
Large *raw* vegetable salad and avocado or beans (garbanzo, fava, mung).

Friday
Large *raw* vegetable salad and baked potato or corn or lentils *and*, if needed, one steamed vegetable.

Saturday
Large *raw* vegetable salad and brown rice and beans and lightly steamed diced vegetables.

Sunday
Large *raw* vegetable salad and 6 ounces of ricotta cheese or pot cheese or cottage cheese.
and, if needed, one steamed vegetable.

Dressings: Lemon juice and oil and dulse or kelp.

Checking Your Saliva pH

Now, let's find out how we can check the pH of your saliva and urine to see what your acid/alkaline levels are. This is quite easy to do. We are trying to keep a careful eye on these levels to make certain that your body fluids aren't too acidic giving a boost to harmful dental bacteria.

The pH is a scale from 1 to 14, and provides a convenient measurement of acidity/alkalinity levels. Neutral pH (neither too acidic nor too alkaline) is 7, which is the level we should be striving for.

Acid	Neutral	Alkaline
pH: 1–1.69	7.0	7.1–14

To check your saliva pH, you must purchase litmus paper test strips, which are available at most drugstores. These test strips often come with a color-coded pH chart, and by matching the colors, you'll discover your saliva's level of acidity. Your saliva should be neutral or very slightly acidic. If you test below 6.9, you probably have too much acidity in your saliva.

Acidity can also be tested with urine samples, but saliva is a better indicator of your acidity level. If your saliva is acidic but your urine is not, you still should consider yourself acidic.

Also test yourself after eating, when your saliva pH should rise to around 7.8 or higher. If you do not achieve this pH rise, it's a clear signal that you need to abstain from eating acidifying foods.

Always remember, your saliva or urine pH is a reflection of the foods you are putting in your body. In the absence of a medical problem, changing your diet will change your saliva or urine pH.

If you have been following this diet for a while and keep on having an acid pH (the paper is too yellow), try using cell salts. The homeopathic remedy Natrum Phosphoricum is excellent for producing alkaline shifts. Natrum Phosphoricum helps change lactic acid to carbonic acid and water, and is also necessary for dissolving uric acid in the blood.

If, on the other hand, you become too alkaline while on the Fast-Alkalizing Diet (the paper is too green), try eating some more acidifying foods.

Checking Your Urine pH

Your kidneys help keep your body fluids neutral by excreting excess alkalis or acids in the urine. By checking the pH of your urine three times a day, you can monitor your progress on the Fast-Alkalizing Diet. You can also buy urine pH test strips at most drugstores.

Your urine should average a pH of 7 over the course of the day, and should always be within a pH of 6.0 to 7.5. A urine pH of 6.8 in the morning and 7.4 in the afternoon is normal. Start measurement with the second urination of the day, because upon rising, urine contains an unrepresentative collection of acids and alkalis.

Checking Your Blood Chemistry

This is a bit harder to check than your saliva or urine, as there are no tests available that can be done at home. You need a blood chemistry analysis that includes a complete blood count (CBC) and a chemical profile (SMAC). These tests are performed with electronic machines in a medical lab, so talk to your doctor about undergoing this procedure.

TESTS IN A BLOOD CHEMICAL PROFILE (SMAC)

If after getting the results of your complete blood count and chemical profile, you are still a bit confused by the readings, the following table may help give you a clearer idea of what the normal range of your tests should be.

I hope that this chapter will help you determine what is proper nutrition if you want healthy teeth and gums. Switching to more alkalizing foods can bring about remarkable, positive changes in your body.

By now, you are beginning to realize that diet and nutrition are related to whether you have a healthy mouth or not. Always remember that a proper diet can be your best friend in making sure that harmful bacteria do not thrive.

Test	Normal Range
Glucose	80–100
Blood urea nitrogen (BUN)	10–18
Creatinine	0.8–1.1
Sodium	135–142
Potassium	4.0–4.5
Chloride	100–106
Carbon dioxide (CO_2)	25–30
Uric acid	3.5–5.9 (male), 3.0–5.5 (female)
Total protein	7.0–7.6
Albumin	4.0–4.8
Total globulin	2.4–3.0
Calcium	9.4–10.0
Phosphorus	3.4–4.0 (higher with bone growth)
Magnesium	1.8–2.2
Cholesterol	150–220
Triglycerides	70–110
HDL cholesterol	Above 55
LDL cholesterol	Below 120
Alkaline phosphatase (ALP)	50–100 (higher with bone growth)
SGOT/AST	8–30
SGPT/ALT	8–30
Lactic dehydrogenase (LDH)	120–240 (male), 120–220 (female)
Bilirubin	0.1–1.2
Serum iron	75–140
Ferritin	10–100

Test	Normal Range
Hemoglobin (HGB)	14.0–15.0 (male), 13.5–14.5 (female)
Hematocrit (HCT)	40–49 (male), 37–44 (female)
Red blood count (RBC)	4.2–5.0 (male), 3.9–4.5 (female)
Mean corpuscular volume (MCV)	82.0–90.0
Mean corpuscular hemoglobin (MCH)	28.0–31.9
Mean corpuscular hemoglobin concentrate (MCHC)	32–35
Red cell size distribution width (RDW)	Below 13
Total white blood count (WBC)	5.0–8.0
Lymphocytes	25–40
Monocytes	0–7
Eosinophils	0–3
Basophils	0–1
Platelets	230,000–450,000
Nonsegmented neutrophils (bands)	0–5
T-3 uptake	25–35
T-4 thyroxine	6.0–12.0
Thyroid stimulating hormone (TSH)	2.5–5.5
Creatine phosphokinase (CPK/CK)	30–140 (male), 20–80 (female)
Anion gap	7–12
Alpha 1 globulin	0.2–0.3

Test	Normal Range
Alpha 2 globulin	0.6–0.9
Beta globulin	0.7–1.0
Cortisol	5–23
Aldosterone	6–22 (male), 4–31 (female)
Renin	0.4–4.5
Estradiol	10–50 (male), 30–400 (pre-menopausal), 5–30 (post-menopausal)
Follicle stimulating hormone (FSH)	Below 22 (male), 40–160 (postmenopausal)
Luteinizing hormone (LH)	7–24 (male), 6–30 (female), 30–200 (postmenopausal)
Testosterone	300–1200 (male), 20–80 (female)
Progesterone	Below 100 (male), below 150 (follicular phase), below 300 (luteal phase)
Parathyroid hormone (PTH)	Use lab range.

CHAPTER 9

The Best Vitamins for Dental Health

When I'm not rushed by my dental practice, commitments to family and friends, travel, and miscellaneous other items—such as writing this book—I try to maintain a healthy diet. I eat a variety of foods to make sure that I get my nutrients in the most natural form.

I repeat, when I'm not rushed!

Unfortunately, like most other people, I always seem to be in a hurry. So there are many days when I know that my diet isn't as good as it should be. What do I do? I take supplements.

Am I wasting my money? Does life go on without a refrigerator stocked with as many vitamins and minerals as food? Am I just overloading my kidneys and liver when I supplement?

I don't think so. I tend to agree with nutritionist Beverly Mittelman, who believes that the only Americans getting their full complement of vitamins and minerals are those farmers who grow their own food. The rest of us eat food that loses some of its nutritional value as it is transported, stored, and later displayed for sale.

The loss of nutrients is even greater for processed foods. Frozen foods lose up to 45 percent of their vitamins, while canned goods lose about 82 percent of their nutritional value. Both frozen and canned foods lose further vitamins when you reheat or cook them!

Is it any surprise, then, that our nation is seeing an increase in everything from cancer and heart disease to periodontal problems? It appears that what we like to call "food" is in many instances barely sustaining us.

Therefore, I advocate eating whole foods each day—especially organically grown fruits and vegetables.

As we discussed in the previous chapter, your general diet should be 80 percent alkaline and 20 percent acid-forming foods. The 80 percent should be fruits and vegetables, and the 20 percent grains and nuts. And, if you must, you can eat an occasional serving of meat.

As to vitamins, your body needs only very small amounts of vitamins to maintain good health, but it does need them. Any vitamin insufficiency will almost certainly result in some kind of imbalance in your body.

On the next few pages, you'll discover which are the most important vitamins for dental health—including key antioxidants for healthy teeth and gums—and how much of each you should take.

I use the Recommended Daily Intake (RDIs) of each vitamin as established by the Food and Drug Administration (FDA). This allowance is a general guideline, and may be increased if you are suffering from a specific disorder.

I would suggest that before beginning a vitamin or mineral supplementation program, you first consult with your doctor. Vitamins and minerals are not just to be popped in the mouth like M&Ms.

Later on in this chapter, I have included a list of foods that are rich in the nutrients we are talking about. These foods offer you great benefits, and they all come from Mother Nature. These wholesome foods should be your first line of defense against gum disease and tooth decay.

THE FIVE LESSONS FOR NUTRITIONAL HEALTH

I recently read a book called *The Antioxidant Miracle*, by Dr. Lester Packer. Dr. Packer is an internationally known researcher and a senior scientist at the Lawrence Livermore Laboratory in California. He offers five "lessons" for nutritional health that I would like to review here:

1. There's no substitute for a well-balanced diet. Supplements enhance the benefits of food but can't provide everything needed.
2. Eat a rainbow! Each color of fruits and vegetables contains many important phytonutrients, which are whole foods. For example, dark green leafy vegetables contain different phytonutrients than yellow or orange vegetables. Eat as many of these foods as you can.
3. If the fruit or vegetable skin is edible, eat it. Scrub the skin to get rid of pesticides, waxes, and other preservatives or buy organic fruits and vegetables from a reputable store.
4. No single fruit or vegetable can deliver all the nutrients you need. In fact, they seem to work better as a mix.
5. Substitute good fats (raw, unhydrogenated oils, such as canola oil, olive oil, flaxseed oil, and peanut oil) for disease-promoting animal fats, butter, and margarine.

Those Powerful Antioxidants

Antioxidants such as vitamins C, E, and A are quite valuable in the fight against gum disease. In various clinical studies, these powerful antioxidants have been shown to be effective in reversing severe periodontal disorders.

An antioxidant is a compound that helps to prevent harmful compounds called "free radicals," from damaging or weakening the body. It works by uniting chemically with these compounds and rendering them harmless.

In my dental practice, I encourage patients with gum disease to eat plenty of healthy foods, but I also recommend that they utilize the healing power of powerful antioxidants such as vitamin C, vitamin E, selenium, glutathione, and coenzyme Q10.

Beta-carotene (Vitamin A)

Among its many qualities, vitamin A is important in helping some skin disorders, enhancing the immune system, and forming bones and teeth. This vitamin comes in two forms: beta-carotene and vitamin A. Because beta-carotene has much greater antioxidant activity than vitamin A, it is the preferred supplement.

Beta-carotene supplements help prevent tooth decay, heal gum disease, and assist in detoxing the body. When food or supplements are consumed which contain beta-carotene, the beta-carotene is converted into vitamin A. The recommended dosage is 25,000 IU daily.

Yellow, orange, and red fruits and vegetables—including carrots—are rich in beta-carotene. The National Cancer Institute and United States Department of Agriculture recommend that you get about 6 milligrams a day.

B Complex Vitamins

The B complex is a family of vitamins involved in a huge array of bodily functions. They can help to reduce the stress of visiting a dentist, prevent tooth decay, combat gum disease, relieve cold sore pain, and even help to detox the body from toxic metals like mercury.

B_1 (Thiamine)

Thiamine promotes circulation and assists in blood formation. In addition to being needed for normal muscle tone of the intestines, stomach, and heart, it also has a positive effect on energy, growth, and normal appetite. This vitamin is also involved in memory and other brain processes.

The RDI for men under fifty is 1.5 milligrams, and for men over fifty, 1.2 milligrams. For women under fifty, 1.1 milligrams is recommended, and for women over fifty, 1.0 milligrams.

B_2 (Riboflavin)

This vitamin is used to convert food to energy and is involved in maintaining memory and other brain processes. It protects against invasive antibodies that can lead to gum infection. Vitamin B_2 is also used by hormones and red blood cells for growth and development.

The RDI for men under fifty is 1.7 milligrams, and for men over fifty, 1.4 milligrams. The RDI for women under fifty is 1.3 milligrams, and for women over fifty, 1.2 milligrams.

B_3 (Niacin)

Vitamin B_3 helps relieve tooth pain. It also metabolizes fat, regulates blood sugar, and lowers cholesterol. Because niacin causes an annoying flush and prickly feeling, be sure to purchase the "flush-free" kind. Too much niacin may cause liver damage, so check with your physician before taking it.

The RDI for men under fifty is 19.0 milligrams, and for men over fifty, 15.0 milligrams. The RDI for women under fifty is 15.0 milligrams, and for women over fifty, 13.0 milligrams.

B_5 (Pantothenic Acid)

This vitamin helps convert food into energy, and is used to make red blood cells, hormones, and vitamin D. It is known as the "anti-stress" vitamin, something you might keep in mind when that dental appointment is beckoning. This nutrient is so widespread in food, it does not require an RDI.

B_6 (Pyridoxine)

Vitamin B_6 is used in the manufacture of proteins, enzymes, and hormones. It also helps prevent cardiovascular disease. It's been known to boost both mental and physical health, as well as supercharge the immune system.

The RDA for men under fifty is 2.0 micrograms, and for men over fifty, 2.0 micrograms. The RDI for women under fifty is 1.6 milligrams, and for women over fifty, 2.0 milligrams.

Vitamin C

Of the hundreds of body functions that vitamin C is involved in, here are some of its dental functions. It is an important anti-inflammatory agent in TMJ (jaw muscles) therapy and can help the body detox from heavy metals like mercury. It works synergistically with vitamin E.

Vitamin C also helps to prevent tooth decay, promotes healing for people suffering from periodontal disease, relieves cold sores, and is essential for the maintenance of healthy gums. This vitamin is also an antioxidant, and protects against infection throughout the body.

We need an almost constant supply of vitamin C in the food we eat for two reasons: (1) Unlike many other mammals, humans can't make their own vitamin C, and (2) Because this vitamin is water-soluble, the body can't store it for long. These two facts alone justify supplementation of this vitamin.

I recommend that you take up to 1000 milligrams of time-released (it doesn't upset the stomach) vitamin C a day if you:

- Smoke.
- Are elderly.
- Have a gum infection.
- Are pregnant or breast-feeding.
- Are recovering from a surgical procedure.
- Drink too much alcohol.
- Have a cold or the flu.
- Have asthma or allergies.
- Have diabetes.
- Are under a lot of stress.
- Take over-the-counter or prescription drugs that block the absorption of vitamin C by your body or cause it to break down too quickly. Cortisone-containing drugs, some antibiotics, aspirin, and birth-control pills have this effect.

The RDI for both men and women over age fifteen is 60 milligrams per day. However, there is general agreement on all sides that this amount is too low. Many nutritionists believe that we need about

200 milligrams per day, and still others find amounts up to 1,000 milligrams daily very helpful and nontoxic.

Vitamin D

Vitamin D regulates the amount of calcium your body absorbs from food and the amount carried in your bloodstream that is available to build teeth and bones. It also helps prevent tooth decay.

Your body manufactures its own vitamin D from sunshine. The ultraviolet light in sunlight converts a form of cholesterol under your skin into vitamin D, which is directed to your liver and kidneys for processing, and then on to your teeth, bones, and elsewhere.

Food sources such as cod liver oil, canned sardines, and fresh mackerel are rich in vitamin D. As we get older, our bodies become less efficient at converting vitamin D from sunlight, one of the reasons that older people often have fragile bones. It's reasonable to suppose that the teeth can also be affected. About 400 international units (IU) daily is a recommended dosage for adults over age fifty. If you're seventy years old or older, take 600 international units.

Vitamin E

This vitamin's most important role in the body is probably as an antioxidant, protecting our cell membranes against free radicals. In detoxing from mercury in amalgam fillings, this vitamin's mixed tocopherols are highly effective and reduce mercury damage. Vitamin E also prevents tooth decay, helps with periodontal problems, and is used in mouth rinses as an important antioxidant.

The RDI for vitamin E may be given in either milligrams or international units. For males over eleven, it's 10 milligrams (15 international units), and for females over eleven, it's 8 milligrams (12 international units).

The amount of vitamin E that you need depends in part on your body size and what you eat. The heavier you are, the more vitamin E you require. The more fat you eat, the more vitamin E you need. But don't exceed 800 international units when supplementing with this vitamin—above this level, there may be an increase in those pesky, disease-causing free radicals.

Vitamin K

Vitamin K is best known for its role in helping blood to clot. But it also plays a much less well known but very important role in bone formation, thus helping us maintain calcium in our teeth and bones.

Besides helping to prevent tooth decay, vitamin K is helpful in cases where a dental patient is suffering from cavitations and osteonecrosis. It helps the body to absorb abundant calcium, as does vitamin D. Vitamin K supplements are also thought to slow down osteoporosis.

Up to half of your body's vitamin K is supplied by intestinal bacteria. The rest comes from green leafy vegetables. The heavier you are, the more vitamin K your body requires.

The RDI requirements are established according to age. If you are on the heavy side, your need for vitamin K will be higher. For men over twenty-five, the RDI is 80 micrograms, and for women over twenty-five, 65 micrograms. It is safe to use up to 100 micrograms daily.

Oral Signs of Nutritional Deficiencies

Deficiency	Symptom
Calcium	Loose teeth, premature tooth loss, softening of teeth, bleeding.
Iron	A smooth, shiny tongue, pale lips and mucus, sores at the edge of the mouth.
Magnesium	Inflamed gum tissue.
Vitamin A	Gum inflammation, yeast infection in the mouth, impaired taste.
Vitamin B_2 (riboflavin)	Shiny red lips, sore tongue, cracks and sores at the corner of the mouth.

Vitamin B$_3$ (niacin)	Tip of the tongue is red and swollen, but the edges are dry and smooth. Sores at the edge of the mouth. Mouth pain.
Vitamin B$_6$	Sore burning mouth, sores at the edge of the mouth, smooth tongue.
Vitamin B$_{12}$	Bad breath, sores at the edge of the mouth, bright red tongue that may have fissures, loss of taste, dry mouth, numbness and bleeding gums.
Vitamin C	Bleeding gums, infections.
Vitamin D	Softening of bones and teeth.
Vitamin K	Softening of teeth, increased bleeding, yeast infections.
Zinc	Loss of tongue sensation, loss of taste, dry mouth, yeast infections, susceptibility to gum disease.

Nutrient-Rich Natural Foods

There is no better source for vitamins and minerals than organically grown whole foods. The following are foods rich in essential nutrients that can promote dental health. You should include at least three of these in your daily diet—even better, try for five daily and watch your health improve!

Bioflavonoids

Apricots
Buckwheat
Cherries
Citrus fruits
Papaya

Vitamin A

Apricots
Asparagus
Broccoli
Cantaloupe
Carrots
Dandelion
Green leafy vegetables (especially beet greens, collards, kale, mustard, spinach, and turnip greens)
Papaya
Peaches
Prunes
Red pepper
Winter squash

Vitamin B_1 (Thiamin)

Almonds
Apricots
Asparagus
Avocado
Green leafy vegetables (especially spinach)
Millet
Peas (fresh)
Pineapple
Sesame seeds
Soybeans
Sunflower seeds

Vitamin B_2 (Riboflavin)

Almonds
Asparagus
Avocado
Broccoli
Buckwheat
Green leafy vegetables (especially kale, spinach)

Lentils
Mushrooms
Okra
Soybeans
Sunflower seeds

Vitamin B₃ (Niacin)

Asparagus
Avocado
Broccoli
Cantaloupe
Dates
Figs
Green leafy vegetables (especially collard, kale, spinach)
Legumes
Millet
Mushrooms

Vitamin B₅ (Pantothenic Acid)

Broccoli
Cantaloupe
Carrots
Cauliflower
Green leafy vegetables (especially spinach)
Legumes
Mushrooms
Walnuts
Wheat berries

Vitamin B₆ (Pyridoxine)

Avocado
Bananas
Blueberries
Cabbage
Cantaloupe

Green leafy vegetables
Mushrooms
Raisins
Soybeans
Walnuts

Vitamin B$_7$ (Biotin)

Almonds
Bananas
Legumes
Mushrooms
Raisins
Walnuts
Whole grains

Vitamin B$_9$ (Folic Acid)

Asparagus
Beets
Cabbage
Cantaloupe
Green leafy vegetables (especially spinach)
Soybeans

Vitamin B$_{12}$ (Cobalamin)

Sprouts

Choline (B Complex)

Green leafy vegetables
Legumes (especially soybeans)
Nuts
Seeds

Inositol (B Complex)

Citrus fruits
Green leafy vegetables (especially spinach)
Nuts

Seeds
Sprouts

Vitamin C

Alfalfa sprouts
Asparagus
Broccoli
Cabbage
Cauliflower
Cantaloupe
Citrus fruits
Green leafy vegetables (especially collard, kale, mustard, spinach)
Mangoes
Papaya
Pineapple
Tomatoes

Vitamin E

Almonds
Apples
Asparagus
Broccoli
Cherries
Corn
Filberts
Green leafy vegetables (especially spinach, turnip)
Leeks
Parsnips
Strawberries
Sunflower seeds
Walnuts

Vitamin K

Broccoli
Cabbage
Cauliflower

Potato
Spinach
Strawberries
Tomato
Turnip greens

Now that we've looked at the importance of vitamins and how to get them in their natural state, let's move on to the next chapter and turn our attention to the equally important subject of minerals in your diet.

CHAPTER 10

Minding Your Minerals

Like a horse and carriage, vitamins and minerals go together. If you are interested in total well-being, then you can't have one without the other.

The fact is, vitamins simply cannot be absorbed to carry out their various functions without the aid of minerals. And interestingly enough, while the body can synthesize some vitamins, it is unable to manufacture one simple mineral.

Minerals are naturally occurring elements found in the earth. For example, rock formations are mineral salts which, after millions of years of erosion, will become tiny crystals of mineral salts. They will then pass from the soil to plants.

Various minerals are used by the body for special purposes, such as calcium, which promotes strong bones and teeth. As with vitamins, you get most of your minerals from the food you eat.

Some minerals are required in lower amounts than 100 milligrams. They are called trace minerals. Although only small amounts of such minerals may be required, it does not lessen their importance in the scheme of things.

Of all the minerals your body needs for healthy teeth, I'd choose calcium as the most important. Unfortunately, the Great American

Diet of carbonated drinks, junk food, and excessive meat protein has thrown our calcium levels way out of kilter.

Carbonated soft drinks and meat protein are rich in phosphorus. Although phosphorus is a mineral that is also essential for good dental health, too much of it will draw calcium from our bones and then cause it to be excreted in the urine.

Watch out for coffee, too, especially if you drink it black. Clinical studies have shown that nonmilk drinkers who consume more than two cups of caffeinated coffee per day are depleting their calcium levels.

Sources of phosphorus are meat, eggs, poultry, and fish. Make certain you are limiting these foods to 20 percent of your total diet, or you will cause a calcium drain that will take a bite out of your oral health.

Let's now take a look at the six most essential minerals, followed by a listing of important trace minerals. You will also find a listing of the foods which are rich in all these minerals:

Calcium
Magnesium
Phosphorus
Potassium
Sodium
Sulfur

Calcium

Calcium and phosphorous work together to promote healthy bones and teeth, although you must make certain that you are getting twice as much calcium as phosphorous.

Calcium also assists in cases where a person has TMJ problems by strengthening the jawbone and muscles.

Another way in which calcium helps to protect the teeth is by inhibiting the absorption of lead, a highly toxic metal. I've seen cases of patients who had calcium deficiencies, and all the lead in their body ended up in their teeth and bones, severely weakening them.

If your child is prone to cavities, it may mean he or she has a calcium deficiency. In such a case, I would strongly advise that you have your child tested for lead levels in the body.

About 1 percent of the calcium in your body is in your teeth. Another 98 percent is in your bones, and the final one percent is circulating in your blood. It's important to maintain the one percent in the blood, because the calcium there is being actively used for a number of healthful purposes.

If the blood level of calcium drops—perhaps from too much phosphorus—the body will draw upon the calcium supply in the bones and teeth to replenish it. This is why you need to constantly supply your body with sufficient calcium at all ages, not just as a child in the growing stages.

While you can get much of your calcium naturally—particularly from salmon and green leafy vegetables—a calcium supplement of 1500 mg daily will ensure you are getting enough. Calcium citrate or calcium gluconate are easily absorbed forms of this mineral.

Many people suffer from calcium deficiencies because of medications they take or because they smoke or drink heavily. For unknown reasons, smoking lowers the level of calcium in the bones.

Alcohol consumption can also interfere with the body's absorption of calcium from food. The combination of smoking and heavy drinking is especially likely to result in a calcium deficiency. Watch out for the following calcium depleters:

- Antacids containing aluminum may cause aluminum to be deposited in bones or teeth instead of calcium, weakening them.
- Cholestyramine cholesterol drugs can block the absorption of calcium and fat-soluble vitamins.
- Steroid drugs can break down bone faster than your body can rebuild it.
- Thyroid drugs can also lead to bone loss.

Magnesium

Magnesium works synchronistically with calcium. This mineral also helps muscle metabolism in nutritional therapy for TMJ problems. Magnesium supplements can help prevent tooth decay and promote recovery from gum disease.

Even the healing powers of vitamin C are enhanced by the presence of magnesium. Most of the magnesium in your body is found in your teeth and bones.

However, as is the case with calcium, it is also important to maintain the level of magnesium in the bloodstream. If the blood level drops, magnesium may be drawn from the teeth and bones.

Besides helping to keep your calcium level in balance, magnesium also assists in the manufacture of vitamin D.

The RDI (Reference Daily Intake) for magnesium for men aged thirty or under is 400 milligrams, and for men over thirty, 420 milligrams. The RDI for women aged thirty or under is 310 milligrams, and for women over thirty, 320 milligrams.

Many nutritionists believe that the majority of Americans don't get enough magnesium in the diet. Deficiency symptoms for this mineral include nausea, muscle tremors or weakness, irritability, and loss of appetite.

Those susceptible to magnesium deficiency are heavy drinkers with poor diets, diabetics, osteoporotic women, those taking diuretic drugs, and those with kidney disease. Diarrhea and vomiting can also cause losses of magnesium from the body.

To avoid osteoporosis, nutritionists recommend twice as much calcium as magnesium. A woman who is over fifty and not on estrogen therapy may need 1500 milligrams of calcium and 750 milligrams of magnesium a day. Such amounts are not easy to get from food alone. Supplements could make all the difference here.

Phosphorus

Although phosphorus in excess amounts can deplete the all-important mineral, calcium, it is essential for normal bone and tooth structure.

Phosphorus is the second most plentiful mineral in your body after calcium. More than 80 percent of the phosphorus is bound up with calcium in your teeth and bones.

The RDI for phosphorus for adults is 800 milligrams. But the mineral is so abundant in food, there is little fear of becoming deficient in it. If you are going to supplement, make certain that you take twice as much calcium.

Potassium and Sodium

Potassium, sodium, and chloride—the so-called electrolytes because they bear an electric charge—keep our bodies from becoming too acidic or too alkaline.

They also help our muscles to relax and contract, maintain the body's water balance, and carry messages along nerves. Potassium works with sodium to help regulate the body's water balance and normalize heart rhythms. It also helps prevent tooth decay by regulating the transfer of nutrients through cell membranes in the mouth and elsewhere in the body.

The RDI for potassium for people over age ten is 2000 milligrams.

Sulfur

This mineral helps to disinfect the blood, and aids the body in its constant battle against harmful bacteria. It also helps protect the body against the harmful effects of pollution and radiation.

So if you're scheduled for an x-ray during your next dental checkup, I'd head over to your nearest vegetarian restaurant and order a huge plate of Brussels sprouts, dried beans, kale, and turnips—some of the vegetables that are rich in this mineral.

Sulfur is also available in capsule and powder forms. There is no recommended RDI for this mineral.

Trace Minerals

Exactly how many of these trace minerals are crucial to body functioning and in what amount are still not certain.

Some trace elements are needed in such small amounts, they are hard to detect. Nutritionists, however, agree that the following trace minerals are among the most important:

Boron
Chromium
Cobalt
Copper
Iodine
Iron
Manganese
Molybdenum
Nickel
Selenium
Silicon
Tin
Vanadium
Zinc

Boron

This trace mineral is needed for healthy bones—and teeth—and for the proper metabolism of calcium, phosphorus, and magnesium. It also helps to prevent postmenopausal osteoporosis.

No RDI has been assigned. Most people get 2 to 5 milligrams a day from their food—especially from apples, carrots, and leafy vegetables. Nutritionists have suggested an RDI of 3 milligrams.

Chromium

Chromium is helpful in preventing tooth decay because it assists in maintaining normal blood sugar levels. It also is helpful to people suffering from diabetes or hypoglycemia. Many people take it to help reduce their cholesterol levels. The RDI for chromium—best taken in tablet form as chromium picolinate—is 150 micrograms.

Copper

The formation of healthy bone is one of the main functions of this trace mineral. Among its various healing properties, copper is effective in helping to normalize taste sensitivity and for healthy nerves.

If your body lacks copper, it can lead to increased blood fat levels which may eventually result in tooth decay or periodontal disease. Increased fat levels usually produce acidity in the body's liquids, which harmful bacteria thrive on.

The RDI for adults over eighteen is 1.5 to 3 milligrams.

Iodine

The main role of iodine is to help the body get rid of excess fat, which helps to reduce body acids. Iodine also promotes healthy hair, nails, skin, and teeth.

The RDI for iodine for people over eleven is 150 micrograms. Supplementation of iodine is not needed, because the mineral is plentiful in iodized salt. Too much iodine can cause acne or even a goiter.

Iron

Although iron is considered a trace mineral, your body is totally dependent on it. A shortage of iron in your body results in a shortage of red blood cells. Among its many functions, iron helps to promote resistance to harmful bacteria in the mouth and elsewhere in the body.

The RDI for iron for men over nineteen is 10 milligrams, for women aged eleven to fifty, 15 milligrams, and for women over fifty, 10 milligrams. The average American gets about 6 milligrams of iron per thousand calories of food. Women who have a tendency to undergo prolonged diets must be careful that they do not become iron-deficient.

Manganese

When there are TMJ problems, manganese is a nutritional way to help ligaments heal. This trace mineral also contains antistress qualities because it works well with the B complex.

Manganese supplements help to keep the teeth healthier by way of aiding calcium and vitamin C absorption. It not only promotes bone growth, but also plays a role in blood sugar regulation and normalizing the immune system.

The RDI for this trace mineral for people over eleven is 2.5 to 5 milligrams. It is safe to take up to 15 mg of manganese.

Selenium

The trace element selenium is a constituent of glutathione, thought to be one of the body's most important antioxidants. It works especially well in combination with vitamin E.

Selenium is a nutrient that I recommend for detoxification programs after the removal of mercury from patients' teeth. Because it is an excellent antioxidant, it also helps prevent tooth decay and assists with periodontal problems.

The RDI for selenium for men over nineteen is 70 micrograms, and for women over nineteen, 55 micrograms. Amounts up to 200 micrograms a day seem to be safe, but amounts greater than 600 micrograms a day can be toxic. In supplement form, organic selenium (bound to an amino acid) is absorbed more effectively than inorganic selenium.

Zinc

Zinc is important for blood stability and helps prevent tooth decay by maintaining the body's acid-alkaline balance. This trace mineral also assists gums that are recovering from periodontal disease. In addition, it is useful for helping to eliminate mercury when detoxifying.

The RDI for zinc for males over eleven years of age is 15 milligrams. For females over eleven, 12 milligrams is recommended. Anyone who eats a well-balanced diet will get enough zinc.

Whole Food Mineral Sources

I've said it once, but I'll say it again—whole foods contain a huge array of nutrients that supplements lack. You simply cannot fool—or duplicate—Mother Nature.

For a healthy array of minerals, make as many of the following foods as possible part of your diet:

Boron

Apples
Beans
Dates
Grapes
Nuts
Peaches
Pears
Raisins

Calcium

Broccoli
Green leafy vegetables (especially collard, kale, mustard)
Watercress
Dandelion
Legumes
Sesame seeds
Sunflower seeds
Dulse

Choline

Green leafy vegetables (especially lettuce, spinach)
Dandelion
Watercress
Beets
Celery
Carrots
Onions
Parsnips

Chromium

Apples
Grapes
Green leafy vegetables
Legumes
Mushrooms
Nuts
Raisins

Copper

Cauliflower
Avocado
Almonds
Buckwheat
Filberts
Walnuts
Millet
Soybeans
Whole grains

Iodine

Asparagus
Cabbage
Cucumbers
Sea vegetables
Green leafy vegetables (especially spinach)

Iron

Apricots (dried)
Prunes
Raisins
Brussels sprouts
Asparagus
Green leafy vegetables (especially beet greens, kale, spinach)
Millet
Lentils

Pumpkin seeds
Sunflower seeds
Almonds

Magnesium

Apricots
Strawberries
Cantaloupe
Mangoes
Avocado
Bananas
Pineapples
Broccoli
Corn
Cauliflower
Beets
Parsnips
Mushrooms
Green leafy vegetables (especially beet greens, collard, mustard, spinach, Swiss chard)
Soybeans
Lentils
Almonds
Filberts
Pumpkin seeds
Buckwheat
Dulse

Manganese

Apples
Apricots
Pineapples
Bananas
Broccoli
Carrots
Celery
Legumes

Almonds
Filberts
Buckwheat
Green leafy vegetables

Phosphorus

Broccoli
Green leafy vegetables (especially collard, kale)
Buckwheat
Soybeans
Almonds
Sesame seeds
Pumpkin seeds
Dulse

Potassium

Dates
Bananas
Cantaloupe
Papaya
Garlic
Onions
Winter squash
Avocado
Brussels sprouts
Broccoli
Green leafy vegetables (especially spinach, Swiss chard)
Legumes
Sunflower seeds
Buckwheat

Selenium

Broccoli
Cabbage
Asparagus
Garlic
Onions

Mushrooms
Whole grains

Silicon

Apples
Grapes
Strawberries
Asparagus
Beets
Celery
Parsnip
Green leafy vegetables (especially lettuce, spinach, Swiss chard)

Sodium

Celery
Green leafy vegetables (especially beet greens, spinach, Swiss chard)
Dandelion
Watercress
Sea vegetables

Sulfur

Asparagus
Garlic
Onions
Green leafy vegetables (especially Swiss chard)
Watercress

Zinc

Mushrooms
Onions
Legumes (especially soybeans)
Nuts
Sunflower seeds
Pumpkin seeds
Green leafy vegetables (especially spinach)

CHAPTER 11

Those Sugar Time Blues

What dentist doesn't have war stories about the dire effects sugar has had on his or her patients' teeth?

This story, however, goes back to the days when I worked as a psychotherapist. I had a patient by the name of Frieda, who was very difficult to work with because every time she came to our session she would immediately get into her angry feelings.

One day I read an article about diets and how high levels of sugar can cause anger or fear. The next time Frieda came to my office I spoke to her about it.

"Of course, I'm hypoglycemic," she replied. She had never mentioned that she was eating large amounts of sugar, and when I suggested she change her diet, she became very resistant and angry.

We worked on her anger together, and once she changed her diet and cut back on the sugar, it began to disappear.

A couple of years later, when I decided to return to dentistry, one of my first patients was a sugar junkie. It was a very sad case. I remember that when Matt, who was about thirty-eight years old, came into my office for a checkup, he had perfect-looking teeth. Everyone in my office was impressed by those sparkling cuspidors.

Never expecting to find anything wrong, I took some x-rays on both sides of his mouth. What a shock! Despite the perfect-looking exteriors of Matt's teeth, every single tooth in his mouth had decay.

Matt, it turned out, ate a lot of sugar. He drank a lot of very sweet teas and highly acidic carbonated drinks. Matt didn't know it, but he was well on his way to a diabetic attack.

I ended up putting dozens of fillings in his mouth, and that alone encouraged him to change his diet. It was quite a wake-up call for Matt. He had no pain and his teeth looked perfect—until I showed him the x-rays. There were black holes in every one of his teeth.

The moral of the story? Beware of sugar!

A colleague of mine, Dr. Rhona G. Stanley, says that when she sees a patient with cavities, the first thing she does is ask how much sugar the person consumes.

Not only does she want to know about the obvious sources of his or her sugar supply—like cookies and soft drinks—but Dr. Stanley also searches for the hidden sugars in her patient's diet. I follow a similar procedure in my practice.

In the early 1800s, Americans ate about 12 pounds of sugar per person per year. In the 1900s, that amount increased to about 95 pounds. In 1990, Americans consumed almost 165 pounds of sweeteners per person. And the amount continues to increase at an alarming rate.

In fact, since 1983, consumption of sugars and other caloric sweeteners has risen 28 percent. *Health* magazine recently reported that since 1986, the average American woman has added 27 pounds of sugar, corn syrup, and other high-calorie sweeteners to her annual intake. That's a lot of sugar!

More than half of these caloric sweeteners came from soft drinks, baked goods, and fruit drinks. Our bodies are simply not designed for the huge amounts of sugar that we now eat. In addition, these sweeteners often replace fresh fruits and vegetables in our meals.

Sugar is extracted from cane and sugar beets, but raw sugar is banned in this country because of contaminants. Instead, it is refined into white sugar, the crystals of which are almost pure sucrose.

Brown sugar, which many of us assume to be healthier than white sugar, really is not. It merely is white sugar crystals coated with molasses, while corn sweeteners are sugars derived from cornstarch.

High-fructose corn syrup has been processed further with enzymes to increase its sweetness. Sucrose, dextrose, glucose, fructose, lactose, and maltose are all different forms of sugar. Honey is a blend of fructose and glucose and, although naturally occurring, is still a sugar regardless of its form.

Sugar has long been known to cause cavities, but recent medical research has revealed that sugar is also associated with much more serious conditions, such as cancer, heart disease, high blood pressure, and weakened immunity. Additionally, excess calories derived from sugar in food are stored as body fat, adding to the obesity problem we already have in this country.

Impaired Immunity

The ability of sugar to cause cavities is well known by all dentists. Holistic dentists, however, are even more concerned, because we look at the entire body—not just the mouth. And sugar has a very negative impact on the immune system.

Sugar and refined or processed carbohydrates seem to suppress the immune system in five ways:

1. After being ingested, they destroy the germ-killing powers of white blood cells for as long as five hours.
2. They lessen the production of antibodies, which zero in on foreign invaders in the bloodstream.
3. They interfere with the transport of vitamin C, one of the body's most important nutrients and antioxidants.
4. They weaken the immune system by causing mineral imbalances and sometimes allergic reactions.
5. By neutralizing the action of essential fatty acids, they make cells more permeable and therefore more vulnerable to outside toxins.

A Double Fructose on the Rocks

Because large amounts of fructose are used as sweetening agents, soft drinks may actually cause you to age more rapidly. Researchers in Israel found that feeding fructose to animals caused their cell structures to oxidize more rapidly, resulting in harmful deterioration.

This same experiment demonstrated that the skin of these animals began to age at an accelerated pace. Think about that the next time you want to be a member of the Pepsi Generation!

The same high-fructose corn syrup found in your favorite soft drink is also an ingredient in many commercially packaged foods. Watch out for it on food labels.

The fructose used to sweeten soda can interfere with the calcium and phosphorus needed to keep teeth and bones strong. Forrest Nielsen, director of the USDA Human Nutrition Research Center in Grand Forks, North Dakota, studied eleven men who drank five cans of cola a day for three months. The men absorbed less calcium from their food than normal, and they excreted 10 percent more phosphorus in their urine than normal.

In another clinical research study, human teeth were soaked in samples of Coca-Cola and canned lemon juice. When examined by stereo microscopy, all the teeth showed a loss of enamel, loss of gloss, and change of color.

Remember: There are more than 8 teaspoons of sugar in a 12-ounce can of soda.

WHEN DOES 1 YOGURT = 1 SODA?

Think your supermarket variety of yogurt is healthy for your teeth and gums? Well, think again. The "fruit on the bottom" of a carton of yogurt contains up to nine teaspoons of sugar, almost the same as in a can of soda.

Instead of the mostly sugar-laden jam that you find in commercially flavored yogurt, why not add a handful of berries to plain, nonfat yogurt? You'll get more nutrients, more fiber, and better taste!

Hide and Seek

Hidden sugars occur where you would least expect to find them. For example, in aspirin, and in many vitamin and mineral supplements. You can also find hidden sugar in many prescription and over-the-counter drugs. Almost all processed foods are rich in hidden sugars.

Most commercial baked goods—even those without a visible hint of sugar—are laden with hidden sugars. Before you can cut down on sugar, you first need to know where it is.

The best way to begin eliminating sugar from your diet is with the obvious. Stop adding sugar to your coffee or tea, and avoid eating anything with sugar sprinkled on top. Do you drink soda? Reducing or eliminating such an obvious source of sugar can make a world of difference in your quest for healthy teeth and gums.

Most bread—one of our most basic staples—contains sugar. If you're a big bread eater, there are plenty of breads sold at your local health food store that are sugar-free. I think it's worth paying a little extra in order to save your teeth.

How about ketchup? Do you enjoy pouring it over French fries or a hamburger? You might be interested in knowing that ketchup has 8 percent more sugar than ice cream!

After eliminating the obvious sugars, start reading food labels and learn to spot the not-so-obvious sugars that have deceptive names such as cane juice crystals and barley malt.

Finally, you may see products that boast having fruit juices as sweeteners. While fruit juices certainly don't have as many empty calories as table sugar, always keep in mind that sugar in any form is essentially sugar.

Now, let's take a look at sugars hidden—and not so hidden—that appear on food labels and which, from this day on, you are going to try to avoid:

Barbados sugar
Barley malt
Beet sugar
Brown sugar

Buttered syrup
Cane juice crystals
Cane sugar
Caramel
Carob syrup
Corn syrup solids
Date sugar
Demerara sugar
Dextran
Dextrose
Diastase
Diastatic malt
Ethyl maltol
Fructose
Fruit juice
Fruit juice concentrate
Glucose
Glucose solids
Golden sugar
Golden syrup
Grape sugar
High-fructose corn syrup
Honey
Invert sugar
Lactose
Malt syrup
Maltodextrin
Maltose
Mannitol
Molasses
Raw sugar
Refiner's syrup
Sorbitol
Sorghum syrup
Sucrose
Sugar
Turbinado sugar

Xylitol
Yellow sugar

Artificial Sweeteners

While it's true that artificial sweeteners don't cause tooth decay, they are possibly linked to other disorders. Stevia, an herb with many medicinal values, seems to be the sole exception. Some of the more questionable popular artificial sweeteners are:

• **Aspartame.** This artificial sweetener, more popularly known as Equal and Nutrasweet, is quite often found in soft drinks and dietetic foods. It can interfere with production of the neurotransmitter serotonin. This can cause a wide spectrum of symptoms, from depression to premenstrual syndrome to cravings for sugar and carbohydrates that may result in binge eating.

• **Saccharin and cyclamate.** Tests showed that both of these sweets caused cancer in animals. They have since been withdrawn from the American market.

• **Sorbitol, mannitol, xylitol, and hydrogenated starch hydrolysate.** These sugar alcohols claim to be noncaloric because they can't be digested. However, they can cause diarrhea and cramps. Xylitol has been shown to cause tumors and organ damage in animals.

In his book *No More Cravings*, Dr. Douglas Hunt states that sugar alcohols can increase hunger and cause allergies.

• **Acesulfame.** According to the Center for Science in the Public Interest, acesulfame potassium, marketed under the brand name of Sunette, may be a carcinogen.

Stevia

So what do you do if you have a sugar craving? For some of us, giving up sugar is worse than quitting smoking or vowing never to have another drink.

One of the latest—and as far as I am concerned healthiest—sugar substitutes is the herbal sweetener, stevia. The leaves of the stevia plant are 10 to 15 times sweeter than table sugar, and the herb's extracts are 200 to 300 times sweeter.

Research done at Hiroshima University School of Dentistry indicates that stevia actually suppresses dental bacteria growth rather than feeding it as other sugars do.

In a recent article in *Whole Foods Magazine*, Dianne Onstad, author of *Whole Foods Companion*, said that Japanese and Latin American scientists discovered that stevia is also a diuretic, combats mental and physical fatigue, and helps digestion.

But is stevia safe? While widely used without creating health problems in Japan and Latin America, it still has not been approved as a sweetener by the FDA. For that to happen, stevia must still undergo extensive testing.

This is unlikely, because testing can cost millions and stevia as a herb can't be patented by a drug company. No patent, no mega profits. Meanwhile stevia has become a big seller in American health food stores, where it's obtainable in powder or liquid form. If you want to know more about this herb, pick up a copy of Dr. Ray Sahelian's *The Stevia Cookbook*.

I'd just like to add here that we're a nation which is hooked on sugar, and that it is beyond argument that this obsession with sugar is one of the prime reasons our dentists' offices are filled with patients who have tooth decay.

Sugar feeds unwanted oral bacteria and is a factor in many diseases—including diabetes and hypoglycemia. So for my sake, and your sake, learn to live without it!

CHAPTER 12

Fluoride: A Blessing or a Curse?

Almost every time we turn on the television, there's a toothpaste commercial telling us that "fluoride prevents cavities." All these products are endorsed by the American Dental Association.

There is just one thing about fluoride that these commercials—or the ADA—aren't telling us about—that fluoride is extremely toxic! It is a waste product of the aluminum and fertilizer industry, and although it may kill some bacteria if added to toothpaste, studies show that it does very little good when added to drinking water.

Yet sodium fluoride has been added to drinking water in America since the mid-1940s to prevent tooth decay. Today, about half the population drinks fluoridated water.

In studies ordered by Congress in the late 1970s, fluoridated water was found to cause bone cancer in some rats. An earlier study, done in 1954 at the University of the State of New York, found that in Newburgh, New York—one of the first cities to be fluoridated—three out of five children suffered from dental problems.

In nearby Kingston, New York, which had no fluoride in their water supply at the time, only two out of five children had dental problems. A second study was conducted in Newburgh—this time by the New York State Department of Health.

The dental records of children in Kingston were compared to those of children in Newburgh, which has had fluoridated water for more than fifty years. The children in Newburgh, with fluoridated water, averaged slightly more cavities than the children in Kingston, with its nonfluoridated water.

Since that time, political and economic interests have clouded the results of further studies on fluoridation. But enough is known about it to say without doubt that this substance is not suitable as an additive to drinking water. Prior to its addition to water, the only use for fluoride in the United States was as an insecticide and rodenticide.

Besides its links to cancer, fluoride has been associated with suppression of thyroid gland activity, osteoarthritis, gastrointestinal and respiratory disorders, neurological symptoms, and headache. Fluoridation of water increases the likelihood that water will leach aluminum from cookware into food.

The conventional wisdom is that fluoridation of water reduces dental decay of adult teeth by 50 to 60 percent, and of baby teeth by 40 to 50 percent. However, studies supported and published by the U.S. Public Health Service and the National Institute of Dental Research show that fluoridation of water doesn't seem to make any difference.

I agree with noted nutritionist Dr. Carlton Fredricks, who once stated that "fluoride in the water is an excuse for the American public to eat garbage."

I think we'd be much better off as a population if we got our fluoride from toothpaste or even certain foods which contain natural sources of fluoride. This source of fluorine can help protect the calcium on our teeth. With our McDonald's and fast foods diets, we do need some protection—and fluoride does afford us some—but today we're getting too much of it—and in the wrong way.

You'd be much better off getting your fluoride from foods such as Brussels sprouts, cabbage, cauliflower, beets, and watercress, instead of ingesting so much through toothpaste and water.

DANGER TO YOUNG CHILDREN'S TEETH

The Centers for Disease Control and Prevention in Atlanta warn that children under six are vulnerable to fluorosis if they get excessive fluorine in their systems. This condition causes white spots on the teeth, and can lead to weaker teeth when your child grows older.

One study claims that 22 percent of all American children have some signs of fluorosis. Using (and probably eating) fluoridated toothpaste *and* drinking fluoridated water is thought to be the cause of this condition.

While the American Dental Association considers "white spots" a minor cosmetic problem, we holistic dentists feel strongly that the fluoride is changing the cellular structure of the tooth enamel in the formative years when the tooth is developing.

If you are concerned about your child's teeth, I'd strongly suggest that you buy bottled water.

As to our water, I don't recommend drinking tap water whether you live in a big city like New York or a small town like Woodstock, which I call home. With all the carcinogens, pesticides, parasites, bacteria, and viruses in most public drinking water supplies, you'd be foolish not to drink some form of purified water instead.

Chlorination is another potential hazard. It supposedly takes care of a lot of harmful bacteria in our water supplies, but chlorine, itself, is a carcinogen and is often added to public drinking water in potentially dangerous amounts—so don't stand too long in that shower or sit too long in your tub.

A home water-purifying system is an attractive alternative to what comes out rather like raw sewerage through the kitchen pipes. Some home filters offer more protection against contaminants in the water than others, so shop carefully.

Water, Water, Everywhere

Bottled water, distilled water, tap water, hard water, soft water—if you are like many people I know, you're probably drowning in confusion. Let's see if we can figure out what's what.

Bottled Water

I think good bottled water is fine, because it has no fluoride. It's pure water. But you've also got to worry a little bit about those "spring water" labels. Author Larry Laudan cautioned in his book, *Danger Ahead*, that the odds are one in four the next batch of bottled spring water you buy will be nothing more than tap water. Except in a few states, bottled water does not have to exceed the standards of tap water! Standards are higher for imported water than domestic bottled waters.

In this country, the overly permissive levels of bacteria allowed in bottled water are a half million bacteria per liter. Carbonated bottled water is more likely to have a lower bacteria count than the uncarbonated kind. You should also be aware that when you buy bottled water in those plastic jugs, plastic toxins may have leached into the water.

In a recent four-year investigation of bottled water, the Natural Resources Defense Council (NRDC) tested 1000 bottles of water from 103 different brands. One-third of the brands produced at least one bottle that did not measure up to strict drinking water safety standards.

For a selection of waters that the author recommends, see the Resource Section.

Distilled Water

You would think that distilled water should be the safest of all to drink, because all the impurities are filtered out. Just the opposite may be true. The process of distillation can vaporize and concentrate chloroform and some other dangerous compounds. Distilling also removes essential trace minerals from water. For water to be truly pure, it must be double-distilled. Yet few companies do this.

TAP WATER TIPS

When you do drink city tap water, let the water run before you drink it, to flush out bacteria and mineral deposits that have accumulated in the pipes. Also, don't use hot water from the tap to make tea or coffee, since it will be more likely than cold water to have lead or other metals dissolved in it.

Boiling tap water will kill bacteria, but then you must refrigerate it if you are going to use it for drinking water. The water we get from our household taps comes from reservoirs and other surface water. The danger usually comes from rainwater, which washes pollutants into these bodies of water, causing them to become contaminated. While tap water generally gets a bad rap, some cities—like New York City—rate higher in water safety than others.

Hard Water

Highly mineralized—or hard water—is found in various parts of the country, and contains the minerals calcium and magnesium. It can be annoying, because hard water has a tendency to deposit a sediment film on hair, clothing, pipes, dishes, and wash tubs.

Once believed to be good for our health, because it contains calcium and essential trace minerals, we now know that, the calcium carbonate in hard water contributes to the blocking of our arteries and to arthritis, rheumatism, gout, and indigestion. It may also lead to bladder cancer or heart disease.

Soft Water

Soft water can be found in a natural state, but it is more often treated with sodium to "soften it" by removing the calcium and magnesium. The problem with this type of soft water is that it is hard on the linings of water pipes, and can even erode them.

Besides removing calcium and magnesium, water softening removes other large toxic molecules, such as lead, cadmium, and arsenic. But it doesn't remove smaller molecules, such as chlorine and fluoride, parasites, bacteria, and viruses. Only water purification can do this.

Water Purifiers

Activated Carbon Filter

The activated carbon filter system is the water purification system you are most likely to see in someone's home, either attached to the tap or under the sink.

The water flows through a column of specially prepared charcoal granules, which removes chlorine, toxic organic molecules, bad tastes and odors, and colors from the water. It does not remove many minerals dissolved in water, and I wouldn't rely on this system to remove fluoride or heavy metals.

Reverse Osmosis

In a reverse osmosis water purification system, the water is forced by pressure through a semipermeable membrane, which filters out both organic and inorganic particles and molecules.

The tiny holes in this membrane permit water molecules to pass through, but not the larger molecules of fluoride, chlorine, and other toxic substances. Nor can bacteria and parasites pass through.

The drawbacks of this system are that the filtration process is relatively slow, much water is wasted, and the purified water is very corrosive to metal pipes. Filtration can also leach valuable minerals from the water.

Holistic doctor Andrew Weil, however, doesn't see much of a health peril in removing minerals from drinking water by reverse osmosis, since we get the majority of these minerals from fresh fruits and vegetables.

There are many water filters out on the market—many of them inexpensive. They all vary in effectiveness, and you must remember that no filter can remove absolutely all the contaminants found in water.

DOES YOUR DENTIST USE CLEAN WATER?

Did you know that the water you rinse with at your dentist's office, the water used while drilling your mouth, may be laden with harmful bacteria? An investigation conducted by Arnold Diaz of ABC's 20/20 discovered that 90 percent of the samples tested did not meet federal drinking water standards. Two-thirds of the samples contained oral bacteria from the saliva of previous patients. In the same test, water from the dentist's offices was compared with water from public toilets. In nearly every case, the toilet water was found to be cleaner than the dental water that goes into patients' mouths.

The source of all this bacteria is the water lines, the tubing that provides water for your dentist's instruments. When those tools are not in use, water sits inside the tubing and stagnates. Bacteria in the water quickly multiply and cling to the walls of the tubing. When the instrument is used again, the bacteria-laden water goes into your mouth.

According to Dr. George Merijohn, a periodontist who has studied and written about this problem, the bacteria can potentially cause disease, especially in people who have weakened immune systems. This also increases the risk of infections from procedures that expose the gum line, such as gum surgery, root canal, and tooth extractions. Because all these procedures create an open wound, "that's why in medical surgery they never think of using anything but sterile saline or sterile water," said Merijohn.

Ask your dentist what is being done to keep those water lines clean. I use bacterial filters and I urge other dentists to follow suit. However, if your dentist has no filtration system, flushing the water lines before seeing the first patient can help prevent bacteria build-up.

PART
TWO

CHAPTER 13

Remedies from a Natural Dentist

In the first part of this book you became more familiar with the world of holistic dentistry. You've learned that holistic dentists—in contrast to their more mainstream colleagues—consider the whole body when trying to figure out why a patient has problems in his or her mouth.

You've also gotten the lowdown on everything from which are the most effective nutritional supplements for strong teeth and gums, to how to check your own tongue in order to gauge your health.

Many of you—perhaps for the first time—have learned about the potential hazards of fluorine and mercury, a toxic metal we will discuss in much more detail in the pages ahead.

Now, I'd like to mention a few of my own natural treatments for a variety of tooth and gum problems that may be affecting you—particularly my line of all-natural dental products.

I've been using vitamins and herbs to treat various periodontal problems since 1978, and have incorporated all my knowledge into developing a herbal formula that can be used as a gum rinse or toothpaste.

That product line (see Resource Section) and the accompanying mouthwash, are sold in drugstores and health food stores across the country. I'm quite proud of them because they contain gentle-acting herbs instead of any harsh chemicals.

Despite what toothpaste manufacturers may claim, clinical research has shown that herbal products are quite effective at reducing plaque and oral bacteria. Herbs, in fact, have been used for medicinal purposes since the dawn of man.

Herbal Therapy

Ever since the first cave man nibbled on a plant, herbs have been used to treat various physical complaints. The ancient Egyptians, Hebrews, Persians, and Romans used herbs to heal just about everything, and thousands of years later they continue to help heal our bodies.

Today, many mainstream dentists are beginning to catch on to that fact. In the many dental catalogues that I receive, I now see advertisements for clove oil—something that years ago would never appear in the pages of these catalogues. This oil is made from the flowers of evergreen trees and helps to stop the pain of a toothache.

One of my favorite herbs, by the way, is tea tree oil, which is derived from the Australian Malaluca tree. It's an antiseptic and helps gum tissues as well as cold sores to heal. It's wonderful for people suffering from periodontal disease.

There are several herbal toothpastes and mouth rinses currently out on the market, and most of them are fine. My own product, which has been tested by researchers at New York University's College of Dentistry, contains herbs such as goldenseal, echinacea, aloe vera, bloodroot, and grapefruit seed extract, which help fight plaque, soothe oral irritations, and reduce and prevent swollen gums.

Herbal Rinse Irrigation

Although my Fast-Alkalizing Diet, which we discussed in Chapter 8, can help restore the body's chemistry to a more alkaline (nonacidic) and less bacteria-friendly condition, like all nutritional therapies, this program takes time.

Until your body chemistry is normalized through this diet, an herbal rinse can help keep those nasty microorganisms at bay.

This gentle, natural remedy consists of irrigating the mouth with a herbal rinse that is contained within a water jet device. The water jet's fine tip permits you access into the pockets between teeth and gums where bacteria love to congregate.

For preventive reasons, you should irrigate your mouth three times a week to keep your gums healthy. Just make certain that you get into the pockets between the teeth, because that's where periodontal disease begins.

You should also do so after a dentist cleans your teeth. Although a good holistic dentist will have thoroughly cleaned your teeth, some harmful bacteria always remain. That's why you need to irrigate your mouth daily for about two weeks after that cleaning in order to flush out the remaining bacteria.

Almost any drugstore sells dental irrigation devices. Water Pik and Hydrofloss are two good products that I would recommend. Or you may purchase a less-expensive hand-held syringe with a cannula tip that you can fill with my herbal rinse. Irrigate between each tooth for about five seconds. Use a constant gentle pressure, and if you are using the Water Pik, keep a *low* setting (#1) on the device.

As an alternative to the above methods, you can use a rubber tip to gently pack powdered goldenseal from capsules into the pockets between teeth and infected gums.

The taste is very bitter and you should rinse your mouth afterward with warm water. Doing this once a day can effectively combat an infection, because this plant has great antiseptic qualities.

Homemade Herbal Mouth Rinse

Here's a herbal tincture you can make yourself if you're on a tight budget and can't afford to purchase packaged herbal formulas. This tincture is composed of the following herbs which fight bacteria and strengthen the immune system. If you'd like, you may add a little tea tree oil:

Goldenseal
Myrrh
Calendula

Purchase each of these tinctures separately, then mix equal parts—about 30 drops each—into a brown bottle. Always shake well before using.

After brushing your teeth, rinse out your mouth with one capful twice a day or more frequently. For best results, swish solution in your mouth for 20 to 30 seconds and then spit out.

In addition, for treatment of periodontal disease, place a small amount of the herbal rinse in the reservoir of your Water Pik or other irrigating device and fill the rest with water. Put the device on "low," rinsing the pocket between the tooth and gum, spending about five seconds between each pair of teeth. Do this twice daily.

ANCIENT HERBAL HEALERS

Goldenseal

A well-documented antibacterial herb, goldenseal has long been used in holistic dental preparations. It contains the antibiotic, berberine, which in test tube and animal studies prevented the growth of many harmful bacteria.

Goldenseal also stimulates the immune system and is great for sore or bleeding gums. The alkaloids, or chemicals, in this plant also increase the blood supply to the spleen.

Myrrh

Highly recommended for fighting infections of the mouth and gums, this ancient Bible remedy is also helpful in healing bad breath, mouth sores, and all bronchial problems, as it dries up mucus discharge.

Calendula

Well known for its healing properties, this is an anti-inflammatory herb which has been shown in various studies to soothe swollen gums. Calendula, which is made from flower parts, also contains many immune system stimulators, such as carotenoids and flavonoids. In addition, this garden plant helps to heal gastrointestinal problems such as stomach cramps, ulcers, and diarrhea.

CHAPTER 14

Bad Breath and Cold Sores

Over the years, I've done many radio shows on dental health, and one of the most frequent questions that I'm asked has to do with bad breath, or halitosis.

While halitosis can be caused by poor dental hygiene, there are other contributing factors as well, such as improper diet, throat infections, and gum or tooth decay. Chronic bad breath can also be the sign of poor health.

Most cases of halitosis are caused by sulfur compounds produced by toxic bacteria. The sulfur lodges in the tongue, teeth, and between the gums and bone. Some foods and drink, such as garlic and alcohol, can leave their own strong odor on the breath—as can cigarettes.

But because there can be other, more serious reasons for persistent bad breath, such as stomach and liver problems—the first question I ask a new patient is, "How is your digestion?"

In fact, I've seen many patients who have mouths that are spotless, but suffer with persistent bad breath. That tells me that there are other things going on. If I can't find anything wrong in the mouth area, I usually suggest that they be checked out by a physician.

One young man who came in had terrible bad breath. When I examined his mouth, it was spotless.

He flossed, brushed—even used an irrigating device four or five times a day. But he still had problems. I sent him to his doctor for a checkup and he wound up being diagnosed with a serious stomach problem.

However, bad breath is usually connected to a problem in your mouth. It's a particular type of toxic bacteria that produces smelly sulfur compounds. You can often find these bacteria in patients who have undergone root canals.

By the way, should you be getting a "glue" smell coming from your mouth, you may have another problem—diabetes.

Some problems of bad breath are caused by tooth decay under a crown. In fact, tooth decay anywhere can cause halitosis. Gum disease will also show up as bad breath. Particles of food lodged in your teeth are another cause of this condition.

If people are turning away from you when you talk, make certain your oral hygiene program is up to par. Are you brushing, flossing, using wooden gum stimulators, and irrigating your teeth on a daily basis?

It's best to brush your teeth—and tongue—after each meal. First, take your toothbrush and start at the back of the tongue, moving the brush forward. Use short, firm strokes.

I'd also suggest that you change your toothbrush every month to avoid bacteria buildup. You might even begin this oral hygiene program with the cleansing fast we talked about in Chapter 5.

I think many commercial mouthwashes are a waste of time for anything but using them for your car. They contain alcohol and are loaded with chemicals which don't do much for your mouth except temporarily mask the odor. There are also studies to show that the long-term use of alcohol mouthwashes may cause oral cancer. So why take the chance?

Do you ever watch those commercials that show the mouthwash killing off all those bad germs? Believe it or not, you don't really want your mouth to become such a sterile field; a healthy mouth has the proper ratio of harmless bacteria to harmful bacteria.

Instead, use a natural herbal rinse. There are also some Ayurvedic toothpastes you can buy that are excellent for bad breath. These will also get rid of the toxic bacteria, not just mask the odor.

Cold Sores

Cold sores, also called canker sores and fever blisters, annually plague millions of people. They are caused by a virus called "herpes simplex virus 1." This type of virus is more benign than Type 2 genital herpes, which is transmitted sexually and is the most prevalent herpes infection.

Like bad breath, there's a social stigma attached to cold sores, although more than half of all Americans get them. Another quarter of the population has the virus, but never shows any symptoms.

Symptoms appear, on average, about a week after exposure to the virus and can last up to three weeks. This virus stays in the body after the outbreak of symptoms is over.

In fact, once the virus enters the body, it never leaves. It hides in nerve cells where the immune system's protective cells cannot get to them. New outbreaks of cold sores can be triggered by stress, other viral infections, or anything else that depresses the immune system.

These cold sores are very contagious and spread easily through person-to-person contact. So avoid kissing your boyfriend, girlfriend, or your favorite pet until the symptoms subside, which can last up to three weeks.

Cold sores are found on the lips, gums, tongue, and cheeks. Outbreaks are more common in winter than summer, which may be due to the extra stress that cold weather puts on the body.

These infections are more prevalent in women, usually set off by the hormone imbalances caused by the stress of the menstrual cycle. Early symptoms are local tenderness, with a small bump on the lip. This can turn into a blister, with increased tenderness.

There is no sure-fire way to prevent cold sores. If you're susceptible to them, you'll get them. For example, I'm immune to the virus, so I've never gotten a cold sore in my life. It all depends on how strong your immune system is.

You can eat a vitamin- and mineral-rich diet, with an emphasis on foods that make your body more alkaline (see Chapter 8). Also, stay away from substances that stress the immune system, such as caffeine and alcohol.

According to some studies, chocolate, peanut butter, and nuts can also cause the onset of cold sores, so you might want to avoid these foods. Instead, eat plenty of salads, raw and cooked vegetables, whole grains (eliminate wheat, if possible), and potatoes (baked or steamed). Green leafy vegetables are the best source of minerals.

SUPPLEMENTS TO RELIEVE COLD SORES

The following supplements may be taken for cold sore relief:

• **Lysine.** Helps to inhibit the growth of the herpes virus. Take 500 milligrams, three times a day. You can also purchase a cream which can be applied directly to the cold sores.

• **Vitamin C.** Also helps to inhibit the growth of the herpes virus and supports the immune system. Take 500 milligrams, six times a day. Take a nonacidic form of this vitamin (ester-C) to avoid stomach upset.

• **Vitamin B complex.** Works in conjunction with lysine to keep the virus from spreading. Also good to reduce stress, for healing, and to boost the immune system. Take a high-stress formula of at least 100 milligrams, three times a day.

• **Acidophilus.** Helps to inhibit the growth of viruses and promotes healthy bacteria. Follow the label directions.

• **Garlic.** Don't be shy. Take at least 1 gram a day. It stimulates the immune system and keeps vampires away. Take daily.

Herbs for Cold Sore Relief

A variety of herbs can help ease the discomfort of cold sores. In addition to being natural antibiotics, the following herbs also will enhance your immune system.

You certainly don't need to take all of the following combinations.

Experiment and see what tastes best, and which herbs offer you the most relief.

Check your health food store and herb shop for more guidance.

Red Clover, Burdock, Goldenseal

Try any combination of these herbs. Burdock helps neutralize toxins in the system, while goldenseal is a natural antibiotic. Take 1 teaspoon of each (in powdered root form), add to 1 pint boiling hot water, and let simmer until cool. Take 1 to 2 teaspoons 3 to 6 times a day.

Astragalus, Yellow Dock, Red Sage, Myrrh, Echinacea, Marshmallow

You may use any combination of these herbs to help heal painful outbreaks of cold sores. Astragalus is known to protect the immune system, while yellow dock is an overall body toner.

Take equal amounts of each (powdered or crushed rootstock), boil for 5 minutes in 1 cup of water, and then steep for another 10. This can be applied to the affected area with cotton swabs.

Echinacea, White Willow Bark, St. John's Wort, White Pine Bark, Devil's Claw Root, Red Clover, Gotu Kola, Alfalfa, Dandelion, Ginger

Use any combination of these herbs to help deal with fever and sores. They all contain excellent antiinflammatory properties. Not only will they help decrease the inflammation and fever, but will also help relieve the pain.

Red clover is an excellent antibiotic and has even been used to combat tuberculosis. Alfalfa alkalizes and detoxes the body. Echinacea and gotu kola are widely used to heal tissues and promote tissue growth.

Black Walnut and Licorice

Both these herbs are said to bring relief for cold sores. They have antiinflammatory properties and an ability to help tissue heal. If you can get these in tea bags, then hold the tea bags against your cold sores. Otherwise make a tea of them and drink 1 cup daily.

You may also use your juicer and extract the fresh juice of these plants. Mix 3 drops of each with a half glass of water. Take this 3 times a day.

Wood Sage, Chickweed

This is another combination of herbs that are often effective against cold sores. Wood sage combined with chickweed makes a good mouth rinse for cold sore relief. These herbs have been used for hundreds of years to heal bruises and a variety of other skin problems.

You may also make a tea of these herbs. Using equal amounts of the powders (1 teaspoon of each), boil for 5 minutes in 1 cup of water and let steep for 10 minutes.

CHAPTER 15

The Root Canal Controversy

As a dentist concerned with the whole body, I have mixed feelings about root canals. I can tell you that research has shown they may even be harmful to your health. Unfortunately, in some cases this procedure cannot be avoided.

Root canal surgery can often create more problems than it solves. For example, the most widely used filling material for root canals—a gummy substance called "gutta percha"—can eventually shrink to a point where harmful bacteria can enter the tooth and flourish. This may result in new dental problems.

Root canals often require restorative work on the tooth after the surgery. Stainless steel posts are sometimes placed into the root of the tooth, crowns have to be fitted, and other materials used. All these metals pose a toxic danger and can even lead to cavitations (see Chapter 16).

In the 1920s, a pioneering American dentist named Weston Price, who did 25 years of research on root canals while working for the American Dental Research Institute, sewed a human root-canaled tooth under the skin of a laboratory rabbit. Within three days, the rabbit died from the same condition that had made the owner of the tooth ill—proving that the germs continued to exist even when the tooth was removed from its original owner!

As a result of further research, a testing method was developed that shows whether root canal toxins are mild, moderate, or severe. By using this test, your dentist can determine whether a patient should remove a root canal or not. Studies reveal that harmful oral bacteria create toxic levels in other areas of active infection. The greater the concentration of toxins, the greater the color change shown in the test.

The technique involves drying the teeth to be tested, then taking a sample of fluid from the crevice that surrounds each tooth. This sample is then mixed with chemical agents that are specific for interacting with infectious bacteria. The color change indicates whether results are mild, moderate, and severe.

Treatment Options for an Infected Tooth

Here are procedures I use when a tooth becomes infected, but the nerve is not yet damaged. These can prevent having to resort to more invasive techniques later.

Sedative Filling

I usually place a sedative filling in the tooth in hope of sealing off the bacterial invasion by thickening the wall around the nerve. A sedative filling is composed of zinc oxide and eugenol (oil of cloves). It is used when a dentist looks at your x-ray and sees that the decay is very close to the nerve.

This sedative filling works in much the same way that an irritant placed in an oyster can produce a pearl. This mixture "irritates" the nerve of the tooth in a healthy way and stimulates the formation of what we call secondary dentin, which is like a wall for defense.

This wall helps to seal off and block bacterial invasion and keep the rest of the nerve tissue healthy. Usually a sedative filling is successful only when the bacterial invasion is caught in its earliest stages.

Magnets

There are many books that have been written about the healing power of magnets. Right now, let me say that magnets do have the power to inhibit bacterial growth.

According to the theory, the negative energy field produced by the magnet's north pole promotes healing by slowing down bacterial growth. It increases alkalinity by reducing the hydrogen ions in the area, while also attracting oxygen to the affected locale.

On the other hand, the south pole energy of the magnet can actually stimulate bacterial growth. Small but powerful magnets are taped to the cheek skin over the area of the infected tooth, with the north pole placed so that it is touching the skin. Talk to your dentist about trying this healing modality—the results might surprise you both!

Homeopathic Remedies

I've devoted an entire chapter to the benefits of homeopathy (see Chapter 20: Keeping Your Balance). Before recommending that a patient undergo a root canal, I suggest various homeopathic remedies.

For example, Hypericum 30C, taken three times a day for several days, can help to repair tissue damaged by an invasion of bacteria. Chamonilla can assist in relieving the tooth pain which often accompanies such infections.

Homeopathic remedies can be found at almost any health food store, and there are sufficient books on the subject. Even pharmacies are beginning to carry these little bottles filled with this powerful natural medicine.

Acupressure

This is a healing modality I often use to help relieve the pain of an aching tooth. It involves applying pressure to various pressure points on the hand. These pressure points have meridians or energy channels that are linked to everything from the teeth to the toes, and by massaging them it often helps pain go away.

You can try it by placing pressure on the bottom of the "vee" formed by your index finger and thumb on the top of your hand.

Stimulating that point on the side of the body where the toothache is may provide you with relief from the pain. However, if the infection is severe, this may not be an effective method.

Ozone Therapy

Ozone is injected into the root canal before the final filling is placed. Ozone is a form of oxygen that is regarded as highly antibacterial. It is an excellent method of getting rid of bacteria after all the regular cleaning techniques have been used. Ozone can also be injected into abscesses, and reports I have seen state that all types of infections have been healed.

Resonant Frequency Therapy

The theory behind Resonant Frequency Therapy (RFT) is that certain sound waves can actually zap harmful bacteria. Believe it or not, all I can tell you is that patients who have undergone this simple treatment report less tooth pain afterward.

RFT works through a machine called the Rife Device. This device was created in the late 1930s. Back then, the sound frequency bands produced by the device were used to try and heal cancer patients, with some success.

Sound frequency therapy eventually went out of fashion, and has not been used much in the past fifty years. Nowadays, however, it is experiencing a resurgence of popularity.

Proponents of this treatment—myself included—believe that every living creature has its own unique vibrational energy field. Through the use of this device, it may be possible to find the right frequency to similarly zap bacteria or viruses. Researchers say they have discovered frequencies that affect six different types of oral bacteria. They further claim it may soon be possible to tune in to the frequency of any organism and bombard it into oblivion.

I have used RFT before or after doing root canal work. You don't hear anything when the machine is working—it's just an electronic frequency. There's absolutely no discomfort involved in this procedure, which usually takes about 30 minutes.

Pulpotomy

This procedure involves cutting off part of the nerve tissue and trying to save the remainder of the nerve. If the bacterial infection has just begun to invade the nerve tissue, the top of the nerve can be surgically removed and a dressing of calcium compounds placed in the nerve chamber.

Pulpotomies have been in use for many years in children's dentistry. But because adult nerve tissue is not as resilient as a child's, this technique has met with less success when applied to adults.

Root Canal Surgery or Tooth Extraction?

This decision is up to you. Extractions and surgery are treatments of the last resort. But if the infection in your tooth has progressed to a point where your nerve is damaged, this is a choice you face.

Although root canals have been an accepted treatment for more than a hundred years, keep in mind that this surgery can lead to further infection and a return trip to the dental chair.

Many dentists—holistic as well as mainstream—believe that it's safer to extract a diseased tooth than undergo root canals. I consider this kind of thinking radical, since not everyone experiences ill effects from root canal surgery. I would think twice before deciding upon extraction.

What Is Root Canal?

Let's pause for a moment and learn exactly what a root canal is. Simply explained, it's a way of burrowing into a bacteria-infected tooth, digging out the decay and infection, and then sealing the tooth shut.

By removing the infected tissue within the tooth, "sterilizing" the canal of the tooth, and then sealing it off, some dentists hope they can prevent the spread of infection. Unfortunately, this scenario doesn't always work. Patients with impaired immune systems are unable to keep the harmful bacteria contained.

Not only do some of them manage to survive the sterilization process, but once sealed off from all oxygen and the outside world, these harmful bacteria do a remarkable thing: they begin to metabolize differently.

They change from aerobic, or oxygen-breathing creatures, to anaerobic ones, and start producing extremely toxic waste products microscopic enough to filter out of the teeth and into the bloodstream.

Once these toxins are released, some researchers suspect they may eventually contribute to such autoimmune diseases as arthritis, multiple sclerosis, lupus, and suppression of bone marrow.

Unfortunately, once you have a root canal, there is little your immune system can do to fight back. Since these harmful microorganisms are so successfully sealed in, the body's bacteria-fighting white blood cells are simply too big to squeeze into that space.

What Happens in Root Canal Surgery?

After x-raying and numbing the area around the infected tooth, the endodontist (specialist in root canal surgery) or dentist drills a hole through the tooth and removes the pulp from the pulp chamber and root canals. These hollow areas occur within the tooth dentin and contain nerves, blood, and tissue.

The chamber and canals are cleaned by filing their sides. The dentist flushes the chamber and canals with an antibacterial solution. Some dentists fill the pulp chamber and root canals immediately, while others wait for a second appointment.

The permanent filling material which is used is called "gutta percha," a sticky substance made from a rubber tree. Next, the dentist will most likely use an amalgam, or silver, filling and crown to strengthen the root-canaled tooth.

When Root Canal Is the Only Alternative

Despite the risks involved, the fact is that once a patient's tooth is severely decayed and the nerve attacked, a root canal is necessary. The only difference between how I treat a root canal and how my more conventional colleagues do, is my choice of a sealant.

I use a product only recently approved in the United States called BioCalex, a nontoxic, calcium-based filler. It has been successfully used for years in Europe.

This calcium oxide, when placed in a tooth, actually expands to fill and seal the root canal. It is also naturally antibacterial. Once in the tooth, it undergoes a chemical change and forms calcium hydroxide and calcium carbonate. This results in a material that is very alkaline, and as you now know, harmful bacteria despise this type of environment.

In a 1990 Italian study, researchers found that not only does calcium oxide effectively sterilize the root canal, but that it is able to specifically target anaerobic forms of bacteria.

Karen's Story

One patient I can recall who benefited from the use of calcium oxide fillings was Karen, a business owner in her late forties.

Karen had a serious problem. About a year previously, she had gotten the flu and had never managed to completely free herself of its symptoms. When she visited her dentist for a routine checkup, Karen was told that she needed two root canals and a crown.

A few weeks after the surgery was completed, Karen had what seemed to her to be another attack of the flu. She couldn't swallow, had trouble breathing, experienced a lack of stamina, and her glands were swollen.

As an athletic person who took care of her body and who had never had a protracted illness before this flu bug, Karen became really concerned. She questioned her dentist about materials and procedures used in her root canal, but got no satisfactory answer. Instead, the dentist gave her an antibiotic, which began to cause cramps in her upper back.

Upset, she went to her physician for a full checkup. Her lab tests found nothing wrong, but her symptoms persisted. At this point, her physician diagnosed fibromyalgia, a disease of the nervous system.

Karen, however, felt that she needed more information. She read about fibromyalgia, did deep breathing exercises, and went on a vitamin and herb program. But her condition did not improve.

At this point, Karen was becoming desperate. She heard of a friend who had had a similar problem that disappeared after a root-canaled tooth was extracted. Karen returned to her dentist and demanded a complete new set of dental x-rays.

Because a set of x-rays had been taken less than two years earlier, her dentist advised against it. Karen insisted. This time an abscess showed up under an old root canal.

Convinced now that her teeth were poisoning her, she came to my office to have nontoxic root canal done using calcium oxide. Her treatment went smoothly. I took out all her fillings from her canals and replaced them with the calcium compound.

A month later Karen came by the office to update me on her progress. Her breathing and swallowing problems were gone, as was 70 percent of her pain.

She urged me to mention her case in this book, because she felt that a large number of people are misdiagnosed with chronic fatigue, fibromyalgia, environmental illness, or something else, when they really have a dental infection.

"Teeth are like no-man's-land," Karen told me. "Doctors don't go near them and dentists don't think about how they affect your general health."

Marcia's Story

Marcia also had success with calcium oxide fillings, because of their antibacterial quality. The forty-seven-year-old bank manager came to see me for a checkup because her mouth had a "funny taste."

She said it tasted like she had eaten "something rotten." Karen's medical history revealed that she was feeling tired all the time and had very recently developed some allergies to food and pollen.

After examining her, I told Karen that one tooth was very badly infected. First, we tried various herbal and other approaches. But when her condition did not improve, I suggested that she get a root canal. The only other option was extracting the tooth. I used calcium oxide for the root canal filling and everything went well with the procedure.

About two months later, I got a call from Marcia. She said she had a much greater amount of energy these days and her allergies were decreasing. I explained that this was probably because the toxins from the infected tooth were no longer present.

At this point you may reasonably ask, "why more dentists don't use BioCalex if it's so good?" The answer is, the use of calcium oxide fillings makes conventional dentists uncomfortable on two counts:

First, they have been trained to pack fillings tightly into teeth, while calcium oxide fillings expand, and should not be made so compact. Secondly, calcium oxide fillings don't show up as well on dental x-rays, thereby depriving dentists of a convenient way to check their work.

Preventing Root Canals

Root canal surgery can be prevented only when bacteria still have not invaded the nerve. Otherwise, it's too late. At this earlier stage, the first thing I do is see if I can shore up the patient's immune system to combat the infection.

If you were to come into my office with a pain in your tooth, I'd take an x-ray and determine whether the decay was into the nerve. If not, I'd utilize every alternative healing technique I could muster, from nutritional supplements and homeopathic remedies to magnetic therapy.

Next, I'd apply a sedative dressing to "stimulate" the tooth and cause the "wall" around the nerve to grow thicker. This thicker wall becomes a barrier against the further spread of the harmful bacteria.

If you were experiencing pain or discomfort, I might also use some acupressure techniques to bring relief. Should all these natural methods fail, I would administer painkillers and then discuss the pros and cons of root canal surgery.

Some patients want to know whether they should remove all their root canals. Many holistic dentists believe they should do so, but I am not certain that I agree.

Much of it depends on a patient's state of health. Let's say you're a fifty-year-old man or woman coming into my office and are in perfect health. You have three or four root canals in your mouth, and you want to know if you should get them removed and replaced by nontoxic substances.

I first ask how the patient feels. If the answer is "fine," then I'll advise leaving their teeth alone! But if they have a serious illness, I'd suggest they give careful thought about doing so.

In such a situation, your immune system is most likely in deep distress and the toxins in your mouth from the root canals are probably contributing to your health problems.

But even with such patients, I first advise that they build up their immune systems with healthy foods, vitamins, and minerals.

When Bad Things Happen to Smart People

Dr. Boyd Haley is a professor of medicinal chemistry and biochemistry at the College of Pharmacy of the University of Kentucky and a well-known researcher in his field. One day, he was faced with the root canal problem as a parent rather than as a researcher.

His daughter had been chronically ill for years, and visits to doctor after doctor had proved fruitless. No one could find the cause of the illness or a way to help his child.

Dr. Haley happened to meet a holistic dentist, who suggested that his daughter have her root-canaled teeth and mercury-loaded amalgam fillings removed. In desperation, Dr. Haley went and did so. His whole life suddenly turned around as his daughter's health began to improve.

Like most people, Dr. Haley had no idea that mercury was part of the filling material that most dentists use. (I'll have much more to say about this controversial issue in the pages to come.)

Upon investigating the facts, he was astounded that this was happening in present-day America, because, as he so aptly put it, "High school chemistry would demonstrate that mercury will leave the filling and enter the body." It just evaporates right out.

After removal of her mercury fillings and root-canaled teeth, his daughter's health not only improved, but she eventually made a full recovery without the use of any other medications. Naturally, the curiosity of her scientist father was aroused.

In preliminary research, he identified various toxins in root-canaled teeth by using radioactive probes. "The data collected indicated that not all root-canaled teeth showed obvious toxicity," Dr. Haley said. "About 75 percent did, and about 25 percent of these were extremely toxic."

What can I say except that in the future, you need to take better care of your general health in addition to your mouth. Preventive care is always the key.

A Final Word

At the present time, about 25 million root canal procedures are being done annually in the United States. However, many holistic dentists advocate removing a tooth rather than having root canal therapy.

As I've already mentioned, this seems to be a radical approach to the problem, since some studies show that only about 20 percent of root canals result in other health problems.

Dr. Weston Price, whom we mentioned earlier, concluded that many people with root-canaled teeth have absolutely no health problems as a result. He believed that their immune systems were able to handle the stress that the toxins from their root-canaled teeth placed on their bodies.

So, should you need root canal work done, don't become fearful that you may eventually be the candidate for a terrible fate. Instead, think positively.

Work on keeping your immune system healthy and your mind calm. Back in the 1920s, when Price did his research, few supplements were available. Today, if you need root canal therapy, you can make certain that your immune system is kept at a peak level not only by eating properly, but also by supplementing.

NUTRIENTS THAT BOOST THE IMMUNE SYSTEM

Nutrient	Dosage	Purpose
L-Arginine	Follow label	Enhances the immune system. Don't take with milk. For better absorption, take with 50 mg vitamin B_6 and 100 mg vitamin C.
Bovine colostrum	Follow label	Enhances the immune system. Contains immunoglobulins and antibody-stimulating factors.
Coenzyme Q10	100 mg a day	Supports the immune system.
Evening primrose oil	Follow label	Essential fatty acids for immune system.
Garlic	Two capsules three times a day	Stimulates the immune system.
Glutathione	Follow label	Protects immune system cells.
Kelp	2000–3000 mg a day	Rich in minerals needed by the immune system.
Manganese	2 mg a day	Needed by immune system.
L-Ornithine	Follow label	Enhances the immune system. Don't take with milk. For better absorption, take with 50 mg vitamin B_6 and 100 mg vitamin C.
Pycnogenol®	Follow label	Enhances immune system. Take with meals.
Quercetin	Follow label	Increases immunity. More effective when taken with bromelain.

Shiitake mushroom	Follow label	Builds immunity, as also do maitake and reishi mushrooms.
Vitamin A plus natural carotenoid complex	10,000 IU a day	Needed by immune system.
Vitamin B complex	100 mg, three times a day, with meals	Helps immune system function under stress.
Vitamin C with bioflavonoids	5000–20,000 mg a day, in divided doses	Important antioxidant.
Vitamin E	400 IU a day	Important antioxidant.
Zinc chelate	50 mg a day, maximum	Needed by immune system.

HERBS THAT BOOST THE IMMUNE SYSTEM

These herbs can be taken as teas. A general rule of thumb is to use 3 teaspoons of herbs per cup of boiling water. For more information, check with your herbalist.

Antioxidant Herbs

Astragalus	Alkalizes and detoxifies the body.
Hawthorn extract	Alkalizes the body.
Pau d'arco	Natural antifungal agent.
White willow	Alleviates pain as well and enhances the immune system.

Enzyme Therapy Herbs

Goldenseal	Cure-all type of herb that strengthens the immune system.
Green tea	Strengthens the immune system.
Licorice root	Supports the body's immune system. Don't use if you have high blood pressure.
Milk thistle seed extract	Excellent antioxidant.
Oregon grape	An immune system booster.

Tonic Herbs

Bee propolis	Boosts the immune system.
Echinacea root	A natural antibiotic.
Ginseng	Enhances the immune system.
Royal jelly	A good immune system booster.

CHAPTER 16

Cavitation—The Hole in Your Jaw

Sometimes, people who have had a tooth extracted later complain of "phantom" tooth pain. Their missing tooth hurts, as if it were still sitting there in its socket. Or they may feel pain in a healthy tooth next to the empty space of the extracted tooth.

Unfortunately for them, this may cause some dentists to decide that the healthy tooth needs root canal work. They'll take an x-ray, not see anything, and immediately think that it's a nerve problem.

The cause of that pain, however, may very well be something called a *cavitation*. This is a hole in the jaw where a tooth has been removed, and the area is not properly cleaned out.

Instead, some surrounding gum material is usually left behind and that leftover membrane may fool the body into thinking that the tooth is still in the mouth. But the new bone has not filled in properly. This is when a cavitation appears—a mushy depression (a cavity) subject to infection and the death of surrounding bone tissue.

Cavitations can result in dead bone material—*osteonecrosis*—and other debris collecting at the site which may produce nerve pain (neuralgia), usually in the head, face, neck, or shoulders. Osteonecrosis can also result in low back pain, pain in the groin or legs, and other disorders.

Cavitation is a relatively new term in dentistry which is still not talked about much in dental schools. As a result, not all dentists are aware of the problem. I wasn't taught anything about it when I went to dental school, and that still is generally the case.

Another problem is that cavitations often do not appear on x-rays. Neither do cavitations show up well on all CAT scans, magnetic resonance imaging (MRI), or radioisotope bone scans with one exception—a new sonogram diagnostic device called the Cavitat, which has had much initial success in detecting this condition.

So, when a patient comes in complaining about tooth pain but nothing shows up on the x-ray, it becomes a judgment call for the dentist, who may decide to do root canal work.

I, personally, must see something conclusive on the x-rays before I recommend any kind of surgery. Otherwise, I'll treat my patient with homeopathic remedies. If the pain doesn't go away, then it probably is an infected nerve, and I'll go to work on it.

When I need to extract a tooth, I make certain that the remaining area is thoroughly cleaned of all debris, including any remaining ligament and bone debris.

If I don't, I know that I may be paving the way for a future cavitation. Other than such a thorough cleaning, there's not much else that can be done. Ultimately, the proper healing of the area is up to Mother Nature.

FACTS ABOUT CAVITATIONS

- Most people who suffer cavitation symptoms are between ages forty and sixty, but cases have occurred in people as young as eighteen and old as eighty-four.
- Slightly more women than men have cavitations.
- A cavitation can occur at the site of any tooth socket in either the upper or lower jawbones, but the sites of the third molar are most frequently affected.
- For unknown reasons, the right side of the face is nearly twice as likely to be affected as the left side.
- One in three people with cavitations have more than one.

- One in ten people with cavitations have them on both sides of the upper and lower jawbones.
- Most people have a cavitation for six years before it is diagnosed properly.

Dig We Must

Patients often come to me who have had extractions done. They tell me that they don't feel well. I've taken out their mercury fillings, I've replaced their root canal, and their doctor has checked them out physically. Still, they tell me they're having discomfort in their mouth.

This is when I begin looking for cavitations. I will open the site where the tooth was extracted and start cleaning it out thoroughly, using a technique a colleague of mine, author and holistic dentist Mark A. Breiner, suggests.

First, he injects a special homeopathic medication called "Sanum Remedies" into the cavitation. This remedy is formulated to reduce bacterial infections. Then, he applies a modified form of low-level laser therapy to the area.

Low-level laser therapy works because bacteria, which are darker than the bone, will absorb light faster than the lighter-colored bone. The laser light then destroys these bacteria.

Only if these two methods should fail to relieve the problem does he resort to surgically opening the cavitation and cleaning it out.

Neuralgia and Facial Pain

Trigeminal neuralgia (TN) is believed to be the worst physical pain a human can feel. It's a severe pain that lasts for several seconds and is usually felt along the jawbone. It has sometimes been described as a lightning flash of pain that doubles a person up. Only high doses of narcotics can deaden the pain.

According to conventional medicine, TN has no known cause, and only drugs can relieve the pain. However, Dr. Jerry Bouquot, former head of oral pathology at the University of West Virginia, found that 70 percent of the people with cases of such neuralgia found an end to their pain when they had cavitations corrected. Obviously, you should consult your physician for any type of lingering discomfort.

Not all cavitations result in symptoms of TN. They have caused other problems, as well, such as chronic migraine headaches. Research is currently underway into the exact relationship between cavitations, osteonecrosis, and various forms of neuralgia, or nerve pain.

In a recent radio interview with Michael G. LaMarche, a dentist from Lake Stevens, Washington, local radio talk show host Laura Lee asked how we can feel pain in a bone.

Dr. LaMarche replied that people can fall and break a hip without feeling any pain, as hipbones don't possess sensory nerve endings.

The jawbone, he went on to explain, is the only bone possessing sensory nerve endings that can transmit pain. He gave the following examples of the number of nerve endings attached to various kinds of teeth, explaining that the large number of nerve endings are due to the fact that the teeth are attached to the head and neck sensory system.

Tooth	Nerve Fibers Attached
Molar	15,000
Bicuspid	12,000
Incisor	9,000

According to Dr. LaMarche, when a cavitation forms, the enzymes breaking down the bone surrounding the cavitation affect the nerve endings. In addition, gas pressure expands inside the cavitation due to the buildup of toxic bacterial fluids, adding to the discomfort. The pressure inside a cavitation can be four times that within normal bone, he explained.

Cavitation and Multiple Sclerosis

Dr. LaMarche is also investigating whether cavitations play a role in multiple sclerosis. He suspects that as the destructive enzymes in the empty hole break down the bone around the cavitation, they eat down and wound the nerves, causing the disintegration of the myelin sheath that protects nerves like insulation protects electric wires.

This enzyme attack, he believes, then somehow triggers an autoimmune reaction, which can lead to multiple sclerosis.

Should I Leave My Teeth Alone?

While cavitations may result in a variety of physical symptoms, this does not necessarily mean that you should be afraid of having a tooth or teeth extracted if your dentist believes such treatment is necessary. Tell your dentist that you expect a thorough cleaning of the excavation area, to prevent development of a cavitation problem.

As a holistic dentist, I am also concerned about what happens to the mouth after a tooth is extracted. In addition to antibiotics, I would recommend the following herbs to help promote healing. They are available in capsule form at your health food store. Some holistic dentists administer these agents through injection:

Olive leaf extract
Oil of oregano
Burdock root

I would also advise taking five calcium lactate tablets twice a day for five days after the extraction. The calcium helps to rebuild bone, while the herbs promote healing.

CHAPTER 17

Are Your Fillings Killing You?

As if there weren't enough reasons for people being afraid to go to the dentist, here's another one. Those silver amalgam fillings in your mouth may contain more than 50 percent mercury, a toxic heavy metal that some scientists believe can be harmful to your health.

In addition to absorbing mercury through your teeth, your body may be getting an additional dose of mercury through wall paint, municipal water supplies—even that seafood dish you had for dinner.

Although research done over the past ten years has shown that in some cases mercury can escape from fillings and find its way into body tissues, there is no conclusive evidence that the amount of mercury released is harmful.

The American Dental Association, for example, claims that the amount of mercury vapor that can be released—especially during chewing and brushing—is too small to cause great harm to the organs of the body.

That view is supported by groups such as the Australian Dental Association and Great Britain's National Health and Medical Research Council. According to Ralph Woods, chairman of the British medical research group's dental committee, "we have to balance potential hazards against potential benefits—that's basic medical principle."

The American Dental Association, meanwhile, last addressed the issue in its 1994 Code of Professional Conduct. The ADA concluded that it would be "improper and unethical" for an American dentist to suggest replacement of amalgam fillings to a nonallergenic patient. I believe this statement was issued primarily out of concern that dishonest dentists will exploit patients' fears about mercury fillings.

When discussing the subject with your dentist, keep in mind that he or she will feel bound by this code of conduct. Fortunately for us, despite the ADA guidelines, more and more dentists in this country are at least becoming aware of the potential dangers that mercury fillings pose.

My own position on mercury fillings is that they should not be used. I have not used mercury in my amalgams for the past twenty years. Having replaced thousands of fillings in more than two decades, I cannot begin to tell you the difference it has made. People begin to feel so much better when a toxic poison is removed from their body.

Opponents of mercury fillings claim that this toxic substance not only depletes the body of vital minerals it needs to ward off a host of diseases, but that mercury toxins also prohibit the body's ability to fight off infections in the mouth and elsewhere.

In some dental offices in San Francisco, there are signs hanging from the walls which warn patients that the mercury in their dental fillings may cause birth defects.

Do you have any mercury in your mouth? Stop reading for a moment and get a mirror. Look inside your mouth. If you have any dark or silver fillings, the odds are good that you have a mouthful of mercury, along with tin, copper, silver, and zinc.

While your amalgam fillings may raise some concerns, they should not be a reason to panic. Dentists have been using amalgams to fill teeth for more than 150 years, and most people who have these fillings do not necessarily succumb to chronic disease.

It is also difficult for doctors to diagnose when a symptom in your body is actually the result of mercury toxins coming from your teeth. So until the debate over the safety of amalgam fillings is resolved, you must decide whether or not you want them in your mouth.

Holistic dentists such as myself have switched to using composite materials to fill teeth. These composites are a mixture of synthetic resins (a kind of plastic) and finely ground glassy or crystal particles.

This tooth-colored material doesn't pose the potential dangers that amalgam fillings do, and they are more attractive. The only drawback is that they may last only about 10 years compared to about 30 years for amalgam fillings—although I've seen them last much longer than that. They are also more costly.

Let me be the first to admit that these composite fillings are far from the perfect solution. I believe that any foreign material placed in the mouth has the potential to cause toxicity.

Still, compared to the possible health hazards of a heavy metal like mercury, I consider these composites to be quite benign. We'll talk a bit more about these composites in the next chapter.

Other countries, meanwhile, are taking a harder stand against amalgam fillings. In 1997, Sweden decided to ban the further use of mercury amalgam dental fillings, while last year Denmark took the same step.

In 1993, the German Health Ministry spoke out about the possible hazards of mercury fillings, and that the country's largest manufacturer of amalgam ceased production shortly afterward.

In my own practice, I have observed various symptoms of disease in my patients—including multiple sclerosis—either disappear or improve when amalgam fillings were removed.

In fact, I found this occurring so often that I actually paid a visit to the Multiple Sclerosis Foundation in Albany, New York, to tell them about my clinical findings.

The reaction was not a very warm one. The people at the MS Foundation did not seem willing to accept this new treatment idea. I'm not saying the removal of your amalgam fillings is a miracle cure that can cause this or other diseases to disappear. I'm not even promising that you will feel better.

I *am* saying that I have personally seen this happen. So if your dentist is still using amalgam fillings, it may be time to consult a holistic dentist.

Margareta's Story

A thirty-four-year-old office manager, Margareta had been reading about the problems associated with mercury fillings and decided to have her twelve fillings removed and replaced with a more nontoxic material.

When she came to my office, I fully discussed the pros and cons of replacing her fillings before proceeding. In addition to the debate over the potential health hazards of mercury fillings, there is also the question of cost.

Margareta's mind, however, was made up. She wanted them removed! In a month's time, and after two visits, I had removed the amalgam fillings from one side of her mouth. On her third visit, Margareta walked into my office with a big smile. "I really want to thank you," she said. "I feel great!"

I wasn't really surprised. Having removed mercury for twenty years, I've heard this many times. "It must be a relief knowing the toxins are out of your body," I said.

"No," she replied. "What I'm relieved about is that my headaches are gone!"

"What headaches?" I asked. Margareta had never said anything about headaches to me and there was no mention of any in her medical history.

"I used to get headaches every day," she said. "I've gotten so used to having them, I don't bother to mention them anymore. But since you took out those mercury fillings on my second visit, my headaches are gone!"

Leonard's Story

Leonard had muscular dystrophy. He needed a wheelchair and respirator in my office, yet he was an excellent patient! Here was a man who frequently had to ask me to stop dental work so that he could get some oxygen from his respirator. All of a sudden, I saw new meaning in the phrase "a breath of fresh air."

I could really sympathize with what he was going through. All of us who have had dental treatment know what it is like to keep your mouth open for a long period without being able to close it. His special need made his dental treatment quite challenging for both of us, to say the least.

I was much taken by his courage, lack of self-pity, and keen interest in life. He had come to terms with his disease and was living the best way possible, with joy and strength of spirit. I had replaced all of his amalgam fillings with composite fillings and wished him well.

About a month later, he came back because of sensitivity in an old crown. After treating that problem, I asked if he had noticed any changes since his amalgam fillings had been removed.

He laughed and said, "What do you think?"

I was puzzled for a moment. Then I realized he had not once asked me to stop dental work so he could use his respirator. Leonard told me that immediately after his amalgam fillings were taken out, his breathing improved.

Some Compelling Evidence

One of the best studies on amalgam fillings I've ever come across was published in 1984 in the *Journal of Prosthetic Dentistry*. Volunteers had their immune systems measured through a T-cell count. These cells keep us healthy.

They then had their amalgam fillings removed and, after a suitable period, underwent another T-cell count. All their counts were up by at least 20 percent! The amalgam fillings were then replaced. Again their T-cell count dropped.

The researchers got similar results in tests on nickel alloys, which for many years have been used in the making of dental crowns. They concluded that amalgam fillings and nickel alloys can adversely affect the quality and quantity of immune system T-cells to a significant extent.

In yet another interesting study, University of Calgary researchers placed twelve amalgam fillings in each of six sheep. Within two months, the animals had a loss of kidney function ranging from 16 to 80 percent.

A 1990 study at the University of Kentucky also had some disturbing implications. Autopsies showed significant elevations of mercury in the brains of 180 people who had died from Alzheimer's disease. These findings seemed to indicate a direct correlation between the amount of mercury in the brain and the number of amalgam fillings in the teeth.

Kenneth A. Bock, medical director of the Rhinebeck Medical Center in Rhinebeck, New York, focuses on family practice medicine. Some of his specialties include the treatment of allergies and cardio-vascular disease. He uses combinations of nutritional therapy, immunotherapy, preventive medicine, and chelation therapy in his practice.

It is Dr. Bock's conclusion that mercury toxicity is responsible for various diseases and disorders including chronic fatigue syndrome, allergies, and sinusitis.

In a recent interview the doctor said, "I approach the whole issue of amalgams in the teeth with the understanding that they are a main source of systemic disease.

"At first, I was skeptical about the amalgam issue, but I have seen so much illness arising from mercury-filled teeth that amalgam toxicity makes a lot more sense to me."

Kenneth's brother, Steven Bock, who codirects the Rhinebeck Family Health Center, is a certified acupuncturist and chelation therapist as well as a physician.

He agreed that "mercury toxicity from fillings makes up 40 to 50 percent of my patients' health problems. Amalgams in teeth impair a person's enzyme systems by depleting important minerals."

During my many years of removing amalgam from teeth, I have often heard my patients say things to the effect that, with amalgam fillings, they felt they had a finger in an electrical socket and now, with the amalgam removed, they don't. Mercury as a metal seems to affect the body's energy field in some adverse way. More research needs to be done in this area.

FROM A GRATEFUL PATIENT

It's difficult to describe a "miracle," but I'm going to try.

My overall health was good, but I noticed a general decline in energy around the time I replaced my crowns for the second time. More root canals had been done in this time frame, and the large mercury fillings were now between twenty and thirty years old.

After undergoing the removal of a half-dollar size benign mouth tumor wrapped around the roots of the two mercury-filled molars, I was having a very difficult time returning to my once-high energy level. In fact, I had very little energy at all.

My surgery was followed by a wound abscess, two apicoectomies and two root canals. The infection and subsequent surgeries required constant antibiotic treatment—seven courses of it!

The surgery left my face numb under my right eye to my lip and half of my nose to half of my cheek, with facial and temple pain on my right side and aching in the right upper jaw near those right molars.

I had learned that mercury is a dangerous substance to have in your body. It is also dangerous to remove, due to the vapor produced by the drilling of the fillings. Not only is the vapor dangerous to the patient—it can also harm the physician and staff performing the removal of the mercury.

Finally, I learned about Dr. Zeines. Although Cleveland is a long way from New York, I felt that finding someone who would truly help me, whom I could trust not to add any harmful substances during the treatment, would make the trip well worth the time and expense.

I called Dr. Zeines, who agreed to do both root canal and crown work, if necessary. On January 27, we finally met. Dr. Zeines looked at my x-rays and said the best treatment would be to remove 90–95% of the mercury—today! He quickly went to work, removing the mercury from both upper and lower molars on the right side of my mouth.

As he was busily working, I felt a tremendous release in

> my chest. It was a very profound experience. It began in the center of my chest and radiated out like a ripple of water in a pond. Then, it dissipated.
>
> I said, "The mercury is out, isn't it?" He replied, "Yes."
>
> I said, "I know, I can feel it." Then I began to cry. I had no idea I had been carrying around this weight in my chest, and with the opening up of my chest, I felt a lightness I hadn't experienced in years.
>
> My energy level improved right away. I keep waiting for that old feeling of weakness to return, but it hasn't. In fact, my sense of well-being has also improved, as well as my feeling that I am regaining the stamina and energy I once enjoyed.

The Long and Winding Road

A little mercury can go a long way in causing health problems, according to the latest research. Since so little mercury can potentially cause so much damage, it's worth while examining what pathways it takes from teeth fillings to its final destination in the body.

Three main routes which mercury travels have been discovered. In all probability, these are not the only pathways mercury can take, but they illustrate how the process works.

Mercury from teeth fillings can be absorbed by the body through the gastrointestinal walls, through gum tissues around the filled tooth, and through the lungs.

Mercury Absorption Through Gastrointestinal Walls

You swallow mercury ions from amalgam fillings with your saliva. These ions travel down your esophagus into your stomach and from there into your intestines. Just as nutrients are absorbed from food by cells lining the intestinal walls, mercury is absorbed into the body.

Mercury Absorption Through Gums

Mercury molecules and ions released from an amalgam filling can be absorbed by gum tissue cells immediately around the tooth or can be transported away by adjacent nerves or veins. Nerves can transport the metal into the brain, and veins can carry it into the heart to be circulated throughout the body in arterial blood.

Mercury Absorption Through Lungs

A person whose cavity has been filled with amalgam breathes in a lot of mercury vapor during the process. Later, with the amalgam filling in place, some of the mercury that escapes does so in the form of vapor that is inhaled into the lungs. Cells lining the lung walls absorb the toxic metal into the body.

Do You Have Symptoms of Mercury Poisoning?

I'd like to repeat that there is still no definitive proof that those amalgam fillings in your mouth can lead to disease.

Many of my patients are in their fifties and older and have not suffered any physical problems as a result of their fillings. Nor are they eager to begin removing them now.

Numerous symptoms and illnesses have been alleviated by the removal of fillings containing mercury, copper, or tin.

Many of these illnesses are autoimmune diseases, a condition in which the body's immune system attacks its own tissues. This happens with such diseases as arthritis, multiple sclerosis, and lupus.

The following table lists some of the more common symptoms of the Dental Amalgam Syndrome:

Signs and Symptoms of Mercury Amalgam Poisoning

A series of difficulties characteristic of mercury toxicity affect the eyes:

- Bleeding from the retina of one or both eyes

- Dim vision, especially after exercise

- Slow and poor accommodation to changes in vision distances

- Inability to fix one's gaze

- Uncontrollable eye movements

- Eyes draw to one side

- Imaginary geometric figures appear in the visual field which migrate in a few minutes from the periphery towards the center and slowly disappear

- A "film" seems to appear over the eyes and sometimes it's actual

- Dry eyes

- A gray ring forms permanently around the cornea (known as Arcus senilis)

One or more heart difficulties may strike:

- Irregular heartbeat (palpitations) occur, often together with anxiety

- Strong pains in the left part of the chest come on

Problems appear in the upper respiratory tract:

- Asthmatic breathing troubles occur, such as a feeling of not being able to inhale

- A "cracking" sound in the lower part of the pleural sac comes on, forcing one to cough

- Red irritated throat shows up

- Inflammation in the upper airways and pleurisy appear about a year after the dental treatment with amalgams

- Difficulties in swallowing are present

Psychological troubles come on such as:

- Severe amnesia
- Constant feelings of tension and strain
- Anxiety
- Irritability
- Difficulty and even impossibility to control behavior
- Indecision
- Loss of interest in life
- Mental or emotional depression

Conditions of the brain appear, including:

- Tiredness nearly all the time
- A feeling of being "old"
- Resistance to intellectual work
- Reduced capacity for work, both for intellectual and physical tasks
- Reduced powers of comprehension because information does not come through
- Increased need for sleep
- Headache occurs about once a week. The headache often is migraine-like, especially induced by weather changes and by prolonged sleep in the mornings.

Neurological complications can come on like:

- Vertigo (dizziness)
- Facial paralysis, usually on the right side that is partly permanent
- Damage to balance and hearing
- A painful pull at the lower jaw toward the collarbone

Oral discomforts make their appearance such as:

- Increased salivation

- Sour metallic taste is often present

- Bleeding gums at toothbrushing

Numbers of other symptoms gradually show up, including:

- Joint pains, especially increasing about a year after receiving the implantation of amalgam fillings

- Pains in the lower back

- Weakness of the muscles with a slowing down of muscular action

- Feelings of pressure, pains, and paresthesia ("pins and needles") in the region of the liver

- Gastrointestinal irritation

- Paresthesia in the region of the lymph nodes under the arms and in the groin

- Eczema or other skin eruptions

Before You Remove Those Fillings

If you suspect mercury may be the underlying cause of your health problems, then there is something you can do about it—replace them with nontoxic fillings.

But before you rush out to do so, here is some information you should be aware about:

1. Since no scientific documentation exists to conclusively prove that removal of amalgam fillings will result in health benefits, you must rely on clinical studies, and the observations of dentists like myself.

   All that can be said with certainty is that many dentists like myself have seen people with persistent illnesses regain their health by having their amalgam fillings removed.

2. Make certain that the dental office where you will have the work done is well ventilated. I use an ionizer near the workplace so that ionized air flows across the patient. The air, which is slightly electrically charged, keeps mercury dust particles down, reducing the possibility that they will be breathed in.
3. The dentist should place a barrier around the tooth. I use a high-volume suction tip that is kept as close to the patient's mouth as possible in order to pick up all the mercury vapor and particles as they are released.
4. Make certain that your dentist uses copious amounts of water to minimize the airborne mercury dust.
5. You should follow a nutritional detox program for at least one week before removal of amalgam. I cannot emphasize enough how important it is to properly prepare your body for a mercury detox program. I will show you how to do so in a few moments.

For those of you who are interested in knowing exactly how I go about removing those amalgams, the following is my protocol. First I anesthetize the patient, and put him or her on the Vitamin Detox Program you'll soon be reading about. I do this a week before the procedure.

I then use a suction device to absorb any escaping mercury vapors while I use the drill to clean the tooth out. One way to remove the mercury is to use a lot of water to flush the mercury out, and the other is to take the mercury out in chunks without touching the tooth.

This is followed by a regimen of more herbs, vitamins—even Clorox baths—to make certain that we are also removing any residual mercury toxins from the body as well as from the teeth.

How to Get Rid of That Mercury from Your Body

There are a variety of ways to do so. Remember: a good detox procedure is never toxic itself. It reduces the amount of toxins in the body, and helps to alleviate the symptoms that may have been caused by the toxins.

The Natural Dentist's Mercury Detox Program

Removal of amalgam fillings from your teeth can get rid of the source of mercury. However, the problem remains of how to rid the body of the mercury and other metals which the fatty tissues and organs have already absorbed.

To eliminate these toxic metals, I suggest that you use a combination of supplements, herbs, cleansing baths, and chelation therapy. The following supplements will help to pull dental metals out of the tissues, assist the body in excreting them, and help repair any organs such as the liver and kidneys that may have been affected by these toxins.

Like the herbs, they should be taken for a week before amalgam removal and for at least two weeks afterward. All of these nutrients come in capsule form and are available at your local health food store.

Nutrient	Comment
Kelp, as tablet or food	Good for mineral deficiencies. Other seaweeds are also recommended.
Glutathione, 500 mg per day	A powerful antioxidant.
L-methionine, 500 mg per day	This amino acid contains sulfur. It is a good detoxifying agent.
L-cysteine, 500 mg per day	Also contains sulfur and has the same detoxifying effects as L-methionine.
Taurine, 500 mg per day	Same as above.
Acidophilus	These friendly bacteria seem to play a role in mercury excretion. One level teaspoon on an empty stomach.
Vitamin B, entire complex	Helps in detoxification process. Follow directions on label.
Gingko biloba, 60 mg, two times per day	Seems to help the central nervous system.
Beta-carotene complex, 30,000 IU per day	Excellent antioxidant. Purchase tablets with the entire complex, not just the beta.

Vitamin C, entire organic complex, 500 mg, six times per day	This major antioxidant works synergistically with Vitamin E. It is also a good chelating agent.
Vitamin E, 400–800 IU per day	Helps reduce mercury damage.
Zinc, 60–120 mg per day	This major component of many enzymes is replaced by mercury.
Selenium, 200 mcg per day	Very strong affinity for mercury. Excellent antioxidant.
DHEA, 25–100 mg per day	Adrenal gland support.

Herbs

Spirulina and fresh cilantro (Chinese parsley) are naturally digestible foods that aid in protecting the immune system. Both help to cleanse and heal and work best during a fast. They can be obtained at most health food stores. Take for one week before amalgam removal and for at least two weeks after removal is completed.

Both these herbs also seem to have an affinity for mercury. Add them to a blender with sea salt and olive oil (cold pressed only). You can add garlic (but of course you can add garlic to anything). Blend until creamy and take one tablespoon with meals. You can also use it as a salad dressing.

Detox by Far Infrared Sauna

A highly effective new sauna known as "far infrared" is rapidly gaining professional acceptance. This low-temperature sauna (100°F to 130°F) employs heaters that emit rays as a special wavelength designed to push heavy metal toxins, including mercury and other toxins, out of the body through the sweat glands. There have been encouraging reports of high mercury levels coming down substantially—in some cases, the patients have become mercury-free in 90 days. More than 300 doctors in the U.S. are now providing this therapy for their patients.

Sherry Rogers, M.D., noted author, lecturer, and specialist in environmental medicine states, "Incurable chronic diseases that were once thought to have no known cause often disappear once toxic chemicals are gone. Since the far infrared sauna is the safest, most efficacious and economical way to remove stored toxins, this makes it a household necessity."

The best aspect of this therapy is its ease of use. The sauna is constructed of poplar, assembles in minutes, and requires no preheating. The low temperature makes a thirty-minute session comfortable, pleasurable, and energizing.

Chelation Therapy

Chelation therapy is a lot less rigorous and just as effective, if not more so, in removing mercury from your body. It's been used for nearly half a century in Canada, and an estimated 38 million people around the world have undergone this treatment.

This therapy is usually done by a physician who specializes in it. His or her experience and skill almost always ensure that you will have no complications or serious side effects.

An ethylene diamine tetraacetic acid (EDTA) solution is injected into your bloodstream through an IV. The acid absorbs and removes excess quantities of toxic substances that it finds throughout your entire body.

Not only is mercury removed, but also other toxic heavy metals including pesticide residues, and various industrial and biological pollutants. EDTA both purifies the tissues and restores the body to better chemical balance.

These pollutants are excreted from the body both through the kidneys and intestines. Chelation therapy is usually given two times a week, with each session lasting about four hours.

The total number of sessions depends on the severity of toxicity and the nature of the toxin. It's also a good idea to supplement with essential vitamins and minerals while you are undergoing chelation therapy.

Because chelation therapy is intrusive, people sometimes worry about its safety. When done by a skilled and experienced physician, chelation therapy has been proven safe. There are no reported cases of any deaths or other harm caused by this therapy that I have ever heard of.

In fact, there are additional benefits to chelation therapy. A 1989 study published in the *Journal of the Advancement of Medicine* reported that EDTA was used on 3000 people who had coronary arterial disease. At least 90 percent experienced significant improvement.

Some people who undergo this therapy complain of headache, mild pain, vein irritation, fatigue, or a mild fever. These symptoms soon diminish. Chelation therapy has been endorsed by the American College for the Advancement of Medicine. If you want more information, you can contact the college at P.O. Box 3427, in Laguna Hills, California.

DMSA

This is a detox therapy that is a bit gentler on the body than chelation therapy because this chelating agent is taken orally. The letters stand for 2,3-dimercaptosuccinic acid, and is known under the generic name of Succimer and marketed as Chemet.

DMSA is approved by the FDA for treating lead toxicity in children. Some physicians who have used it praise DMSA for its ability to remove mercury and other toxic metals from the body, as well as lead.

One study reported, however, that DMSA seemed to remove lead from the body first. Only after large quantities of lead were removed did this acid turn its full attention to mercury removal.

When you go to a physician trained to do DMSA detox therapy, you can expect the following procedure. Keep in mind, though, that individual doctors have their own approaches and you can expect some differences among them:

- You will be asked to supply urine samples over a 6-hour period. Your urine will then be tested for its mercury content.
- Assuming that mercury is found in your urine, you will be asked to take 500 milligrams of DMSA orally three times a week for 4 weeks.

- After a week without DMSA, your urine will be tested again to see how successful the detoxification has been.
- If the physician is satisfied with your progress, he or she will likely ask you to continue taking 500 milligrams of DMSA orally three times a week for another 4 weeks.
- After a week off DMSA, your urine will be tested again. This pattern is likely to be repeated, with dose increases or decreases, until the physician is satisfied that your urine is mercury-free. Most physicians are in agreement that mercury does not occur naturally in urine.
- If you are having amalgam fillings removed from your teeth, this work is likely to be done after one of your urine tests. Since you are likely to absorb more mercury from vapor during amalgam removal, you will be put back on DMSA therapy without delay.

About the only side effect you may experience is a flu-like feeling which should soon go away. Precautions for this procedure include getting a patient on a good mercury detox program, and supplementing with plenty of vitamins and minerals. Most dentists such as myself use special suction devices that go around the tooth to make certain that you don't get any of the mercury in your system.

Cleansing Baths

Cleansing baths are an excellent way to get rid of toxins. They have long been used in Europe, and are effective in removing environmental toxins, heavy metal deposits, and radiation residue. Cleansing baths are best taken before bedtime a couple of times a week. You can assist the effects of cleansing baths by adding more green leafy vegetables and fluids to your diet.

BATHING BEAUTIES

"What's in a bath?" you may ask. Here are a few varieties that can help you rid your body of those heavy metals:

- Clorox baths have been used for years and years, and they work quite well. I first learned about them in the 1980s. A Clorox bath clears heavy metals, radiation toxins, and lymphatic congestion.

  Add ½ to 1 cup of Clorox brand bleach to a full bath of hot water. Soak for at least a half hour and then shower. Clorox, by the way, does not contain chlorine.
- A sea salt and baking soda bath clears radiation toxins and lymphatic congestion. Add 1 to 2 cups each of sea salt and baking soda to a full bath of hot water. Soak for at least a half hour and then shower.
- An Epsom salts bath is an excellent broad-spectrum cleanser for all kinds of toxins. For detoxification, add up to 4 cups of Epsom salts to a full bath of hot water. Adding a cup of apple cider vinegar is optional. Soak for at least a half hour and then shower.
- An apple cider vinegar bath is good for clearing bacterial infections. Add 1 quart of apple cider vinegar to a full bath of hot water. Soak for at least a half hour and then shower.

We live in a toxic world, and few of us can ensure that our bodies remain free from environmental pollutants. All we can hope to do is consciously avoid as many toxins as we can, boost our immune systems, eat healthy diets, and lead healthy lifestyles. We can also pray!

Allowing a toxic metal like mercury to be placed in our mouths in the name of dental therapy might seem to perfectly reasonable people to be a risky business. Still, we all have done it.

Fortunately, an increasing number of dentists are also beginning to see the logic of not using toxic materials in the mouth, so maybe one day this potentially dangerous practice will stop.

Other Toxic Metals

While most of the attention has rightly been placed on the toxic metal, mercury, amalgam fillings always contain at least one other metal, like tin, copper, or zinc.

I wouldn't worry too much about the dangers these other heavy metals may pose, because there is such a small amount of them within each filling. Most fillings contain about 15 percent tin and copper, a trace of zinc, and 35 percent silver.

However, you should remain aware that the following metals have the potential to cause your body harm:

Beryllium

This metal is sometimes added to amalgam fillings. It may also be added to bridges and other dental implants to give them strength and yield better casting.

Some potential dangers of this toxic metal include lung impairment or infections of the eye, nose, or throat.

Cobalt

This heavy metal may cause lung and respiratory tract problems that can become worse over time.

Copper

Toxins released from copper can affect the digestive tract and result in very uncomfortable symptoms, such as pain, convulsions, excessive vomiting, and stupor.

Copper intake has also been reported to cause digestive tract problems and women may experience problems with their menstrual cycle. Copper poisoning can cause problems with the eyes, which take on a sunken, and sometimes cross-eyed appearance.

Some research indicates that copper can toxify the blood supply to the teeth, causing decay. People who suffer copper toxicity often have trouble with their joints. Men may feel pain in the testicles, and women's ovaries may be tender on examination.

Gallium

Gallium sometimes causes mild dermatitis.

Nickel

Headaches, vision problems, and dizziness are associated with nickel toxicity. The upper lip may twitch, sneezing may be violent, and the neck vertebrae may make a snapping sound when the head is turned. Painful headaches are frequent. People often feel itchy all over their body, but especially on the neck.

Silver

Dental silver reportedly causes an array of symptoms, from neuralgia to tenderness of the scalp. Severe backache may also result. Silver may also cause an increase of phlegm and constant coughing. Silver poisoning can cause a sore throat.

Tin

Tin reportedly affects the nervous system and respiratory tract. The head may feel enclosed as if by a band, the tightening of which causes increased pain. Earring holes may become ulcerated.

This heavy metal can cause stomach cramps or a buildup of phlegm that is difficult to remove by coughing. Some people who suffer from tin poisoning report severe nausea when exposed to the smell of cooking food. Excess tin in the body may also cause ankle swelling.

Zinc

Too much zinc can inhibit immune responses, according to a recent study done by the United States Department of Agriculture at Tufts University. Two grams or more of zinc in the body can prompt this response.

I hope this chapter serves as an eye opener regarding the dangers of toxic metals—especially those that may be found in your fillings. I'm not here to scare you, but alert you to a problem to which many people have closed their eyes.

The truth of the matter is that many people today are poisoned by mercury and they don't even work in a high-risk occupation.

Every day of our lives we are exposed to heavy metals. They are unavoidable. What is avoidable is having any of these potentially dangerous metals placed in our mouths.

SAY GOOD-BYE TO HEAVY METALS

What can you do to avoid exposure to toxic metals like mercury?

1. Eliminate or cut down consumption of fish that feed at the mouth of the Gulf of Mexico and the Chesapeake Bay. These two heavy metal toxic waterways are, unfortunately, two of the most common sources of seafood in the United States.
2. Get an air cleaner for your car. It plugs in to the cigarette lighter.
3. Switch from commercially processed foods to whole foods.
4. Try some chelation therapy.

CHAPTER 18

Secrets of a Perfect Smile

There is nothing that gives me more pleasure than restoring a tooth to its natural form and function. When you have a cavity, what it basically does is break down the internal and external structure of the tooth.

You now have a hole in your tooth. It can be a little hole or a huge hole. My job is to fix that hole using natural, nontoxic materials, and then try to restore the exterior of the tooth if it has been damaged with as little intrusive dental work as possible.

For years, dentists would just clean out the hole, take some amalgam, and jam that mercury-laden material into the hole. If a tooth was chipped, stained, or eroded, however, there was little or nothing that they could do about it.

In the past ten to twelve years, however, some new innovations have hit the scene that not only make filling teeth safer, but can also help your cuspidors look a world better.

Bonding

Bonding is one of those new innovations. If there is no root damage to the tooth, it is in many cases an alternative method to filling. In bonding, the same nontoxic resins used to fill cavities are molded onto the tooth surface to cover up small cracks or gaps.

Bonding usually involves little or no drilling, doesn't take much time, and is an inexpensive way of putting a great smile back on a patient's face. Of course, there are situations when teeth must be drilled and filled, no matter what.

Let me say right here that I am no big proponent of drilling. My approach to tooth restoration is to do only what is needed and keep intrusive dental work to a minimum.

There's a new trend in holistic dentistry that may someday be a more viable alternative. We're beginning to use lasers now on very small cavities. They don't really work as well as the ads make them out to, because this technology is really in the infant stages.

Lasers are not recommended for adults who have mercury fillings because they can vaporize the mercury, and who knows what will happen if too much of that material gets loose!

So until laser technology improves, the drill is still the easiest, most effective, and quickest way to repair cavities.

There are also some gels being introduced that can dissolve away some of the decay areas. Someday in the future you'll be able to wash your tooth decay away.

A frequently used bonding technique involves slightly reducing the surface of the tooth to be bonded, so that the added bonding materials will not be evident. Then the tooth surface enamel is acid-etched with microscopic grooves, which help the composite to adhere. The tooth surface is next covered with a liquid-plastic bonding agent.

Finally, the composite is applied and shaped while it is still soft. The dentist uses a low-voltage tungsten-halogen lamp for less than a minute to harden the composite. Some composites are self-hardening. I use lasers for the final curing because they're quicker and yield a better and stronger restoration.

Tooth Whitening

Teeth get discolored by bad diets and ill health. If you drink a lot of tea, watch your teeth turn color. There are no ways I know of through the use of herbs to whiten teeth.

You're left to rely on those toothpaste whiteners sold in drugstores or the bleaching gels your dentist can treat you with in his office. Those whitening toothpastes sold in drugstores are not as effective as the gels recommended by your dentist, which contain strong oxidizers such as hydrogen peroxide.

Some of these whiteners, however, can cause the gums to whiten or peel. If using a home kit, it's safest to ask your dentist's advice on what to buy and exactly how to use it. You'll usually need several applications before achieving the desired results, and you can also expect increased teeth sensitivity after each bleaching.

If your discolored teeth truly are bothersome to you, you might consider getting a veneer.

Veneers

In the world of cosmetic dentistry, veneers are a miracle. They are thin, strong shells of porcelain or composite that are bonded to the front of chipped, eroded, badly shaped, or stained teeth. They are also used to narrow the gaps between teeth.

Before this technology was developed, nothing really could be done for a patient whose teeth were unattractive. Today, veneers work cosmetically in much the same way that false fingernails do. Besides beautifying a person's teeth, they also have a health benefit. It's long been known that people who are depressed tend to have impaired immune systems.

When veneers are put into place, patients immediately begin to smile more. In fact, they really are happier, considering their teeth have just been made lighter and brighter.

One of the things I have always enjoyed about my holistic practice is watching patients discover that their dentist can be their friend. I just love the reaction people have when a dental procedure turns out to be far more pleasant than they had expected.

186 • HEALTHY MOUTH, HEALTHY BODY

However, I was not prepared for Joanne's reaction. She started to cry. With a big smile and tears pouring down her face, she kept telling me how embarrassed she had been about her teeth.

As she left my office, Joanne was already making plans for her new social life. While I am not saying one thing had to do with the other, Joanne got married shortly after I had provided her with a smile.

Joseph's Story

One of my biggest compliments was actually a complaint from a patient's wife. Her husband, Joseph, was the forty-five-year-old manager of a construction project in lower Manhattan.

His teeth were cracked and chipped. A proud man, Joseph hated feeling self-conscious about his teeth, knowing how ugly they looked. I placed veneers on both upper and lower teeth.

About a week later, his wife called. She wanted my advice about a new problem that was making her a little crazy. It seemed that every night when Joseph returned from work, he spent hours in the bathroom, smiling and staring into the mirror because he was so happy about his new dental look!

Crowns

A crown is an artificial cap that dentists place over a real tooth when it has decayed so much that filling it is useless. This cap is a sheath of metal, and the tooth usually has to be carved down for it to fit.

To make a crown, your dentist first has to make an impression of the natural tooth, then of the biting surface of the tooth or teeth to be crowned, and also of the teeth opposite.

The tooth is then prepared by drilling away the enamel and some of the dentin, and then more impressions are made. You wear a temporary crown while you wait for your permanent one—which usually takes about two weeks.

If I can, I try to save as much of the tooth as possible by using the bondable materials I described earlier. Over the years, I have restored many teeth using this method, and I'm quite proud of having saved those patients the needless inconvenience and expense of getting a crown.

I believe that crowns ought to be a last result, and used only when the tooth structure can no longer support a filling. There's simply too much intrusive work involved in the process of making a crown, yet that doesn't stop most mainstream dentists.

Fillings

When tooth decay has penetrated the enamel—the outer layer of the tooth—and is deep into the softer dentin area, it's a good idea to have that tooth filled to prevent harmful microorganisms from reaching the tooth pulp with its blood, tissue, and nerves.

At this point, you have a choice of four filling materials: composite resins, porcelain inlays, amalgam fillings, and gold inlays.

Composite Fillings

We talked some about composite fillings in the previous chapter. As you know, they're a much better alternative than amalgams with their potential for mercury poisoning.

Some companies are putting aluminum oxide or barium into their composites so they will show up better on x-rays. That doesn't please me, because there are some studies which indicate that these two metals can suppress the immune system.

If you are going to get a composite filling, make certain that you ask for composites which do not contain aluminum, barium, or any other metals.

Not all composite materials are the same. The better composites are composed of quartz crystal or some other hard crystalline substance. These composites, of course, are more expensive.

The most widely used resin is Bis-GMA, which forms a hard and stable plastic-like substance, or polymer. The average composite filling will cost between $175 and $350.

Composites have the natural color of teeth, which makes these fillings hardly visible in your front row of teeth. They also look swell—and work well—in smaller cavities in back teeth.

Some dentists complain that the larger the cavity, the weaker the composite filling. This has not been my experience with the composites used today. The only side effect I know of is that your tooth may be sensitive for a while after being filled with a composite.

Although the manufacturers of this material conservatively estimate that a composite filling lasts three to ten years, I have seen them last much longer. I believe they can last almost indefinitely in an otherwise healthy tooth.

However, they can be stained by coffee, tea, or smoking. They can also chip or wear away through chewing or teeth grinding. Another problem with composite fillings is so-called leaking, in which a space develops between the filling and the tooth. New areas of decay can develop in these spaces.

Most holistic dentists are aware of this problem, and when that happens, they use a bonded filling. It's a three-step procedure. The tooth is cleaned and washed out in a dilute acid bath, which lets the surface of the tooth be roughened so that the bonding agents can adhere better.

Next, a bonding agent—kind of like a super glue—is put on the roughened area. The composite filling is placed on top of that area, and shaped to fit the tooth with the use of a laser technique.

Porcelain Inlays

Picture a box with one corner of it broken. We can fill that. But if two or three corners of the box are broken, that's too big for a filling to handle.

In such a case, what we would do is make an "inlay." I can make one out of composite bonding materials—it is much like a filling, but on a larger scale—while the patient is seated there, or have a lab do it.

If the patient wants the lab to make a more expensive inlay—usually heat-cured or made out of porcelain—I first make an impression of the tooth.

Porcelain is a little more expensive than the composite materials I have in my office, and may cause a little more wear on your regular teeth. But the coloring looks very nice and some people are sticklers for that. Inlays also have good strength.

Porcelain cannot only be matched exactly to the natural color of your tooth, but unlike a composite filling, it is also stain-resistant. Also, porcelain inlays are unlikely to develop leakage. However, they are more brittle and fracture more easily.

My own preference is to use the composites, because they can be bonded to the teeth. Also, because some of the newer composites have increased strength, I find them to be very effective as inlays.

Gold Inlays

A gold inlay is custom made in a dental lab and cemented in place on a second visit to your dentist. At ordinary temperatures, gold is chemically inert and thus the leaching that makes amalgam fillings so dangerous does not occur.

However, some people are allergic to gold itself. For people not allergic to it, gold is generally regarded as the material of choice for repairing teeth. These inlays last up to twenty years.

One problem with gold—besides its cost—is that its chemical structure may react with the mercury in your amalgams. So if you already have mercury fillings in your mouth, avoid gold inlays.

Bridges

Missing teeth permit other teeth to shift or rotate, often resulting in a bad bite (malocclusion). This can lead to TMJ problems and even gum disease. To prevent such dental problems from developing, you need to replace a missing tooth without delay.

A bridge can be used to replace from one to three missing teeth. It basically consists of a false tooth attached to the crowned natural tooth on either side. There are new composite materials being used for bridges, so that in many cases metal does not need to be used for the support structures.

Fixed Bridge

This is the traditional bridge that has been used since the days of your great grandfather. A false tooth is cemented to a crowned tooth on either side. The crowns and false tooth are usually porcelain baked onto a metal support. A fixed bridge is strong and normally so comfortable, you quickly become unaware of it. It is never removed.

Bonded Bridge

The difference between a bonded and fixed bridge is that a bonded bridge lacks a metal support and relies solely on porcelain bonds to attach the false tooth to the crowns on either side. As a result, a bonded bridge looks more natural but has much less strength.

However, for a small bridge where one tooth is missing, or where there is not much biting pressure, the new composites and fibercore have much more strength than the older materials.

Maryland Bridge

This bridge, developed at the University of Maryland, does not require the teeth on either side of the false tooth to be crowned. Instead, the false tooth is attached to them by metal wings on the inside surface.

This requires minimal abrasion of the natural tooth on each side. The Maryland bridge works well with healthy supporting teeth, although the metal wings can become loose and require rebonding.

Cantilever Bridge

Here the false tooth is attached to one or—more often—two natural teeth on one side of the mouth and to none on the other. Being neither as strong nor as stable as other bridges, the cantilever bridge is used only when a supporting tooth is lacking on one side.

Removable Bridge

Rather than being bonded to the teeth on either side, the false tooth in this kind of bridge is attached to them with removable metal clasps. Usually the metal clasps are visible and the false tooth is not as stable as in other bridges.

Implants

An implant is a base for an artificial tooth that is implanted in the jawbone at the location of a missing tooth. Rods that are inserted into the jaw are usually made from ceramics or a titanium alloy.

After the hole is drilled in the jawbone and the implant inserted, healing takes a few months. I'd suggest that during this period of time that you use a herbal mouth rinse religiously.

I'd also recommend that you take immune system–building supplements during the healing process. Once the implant has successfully healed, a permanent artificial tooth can be mounted on it.

The good news is that implants have benefited thousands of people. Long-term studies have shown a 90 percent success rate. The problem with implants is that they are in an open system. When an implant is placed inside the body, the metal pins are completely bathed in the body fluids. Even if the implant is in the bone, the bone is surrounded by its blood supply.

Oral implants are in bone covered by gingival, or gum, tissue. Teeth, like the implant, are also in bone. However, while the gum tissue will attach to the tooth, it will not attach to the implant. This means that the bone is open to the oral cavity, with its resident population of millions of bacteria. If oral care is not perfect, these bacteria can penetrate to the bone and cause a great deal of bone loss through infection.

Even with this potential problem, an implant is certainly preferrable to having no teeth.

Unfortunately, if you don't have a back tooth upon which to anchor a bridge, you're going to need an implant. A removable plastic device with clamps that can be clipped in and out is another alternative.

Although this is a far less toxic approach, it is not very comfortable. Most of my patients who have tried them hate them!

Obviously, implants are far from a perfect solution, but until technology is advanced to the stage where we can place in your mouth a little toothbud from your genetic composition, this is the kind of Band-Aid we can offer.

If you are a candidate for an implant, your dentist has to take various considerations into account: the amount of bone available, your response to the materials, and how well you can tolerate what is essentially an open void in the mouth.

CHAPTER 19

From Magnets to Muscle Testing

I have been practicing holistic dentistry for more than twenty-five years, and over the years have studied many alternative methods of healing—from aromatherapy and acupressure, to magnetic therapy, kinesiology, reflexology, reiki, and homeopathy.

Many of these methods come from both the Eastern and Western healing traditions. Some date back more than a thousand years. The study of the flow of energy, or *qi*, for example, has been studied by Oriental medicine since 300 B.C.

These ancient Chinese healers understood, as holistic dentists do today, that there are meridians, or energy channels, running from head to foot. If energy is disrupted along one of those channels, it affects organs all along the line.

Of course, most mainstream dentists view many of these approaches as pure foolishness. It's a shame, because these nontraditional therapies can make a real difference in a patient's recovery—whether at a doctor or dentist's office.

I believe, for example, there is more potency in homeopathic medicine than in many of our most highly touted drugs. Homeopathy has its origins in the natural world, while many of our antibacterial drugs are Frankenstein-like creations of the laboratory.

Peggy's Story

Peggy had a throbbing pain in her lower right first molar. The health-conscious thirty-five-year-old New York City schoolteacher was referred to me for possible root canal therapy, because she wanted a holistic dentist who used biocompatible materials.

Before beginning my physical examination of her mouth, I placed a few drops of lavender solution on her bib. This is a flower essence, that has healing and calming properties. It's not something you expect to smell in a dentist's office, and my patients enjoy it because it helps to dispel the more clinical smells.

While examining her mouth, I noticed that Peggy's tongue color was grayish-brown, rather than a healthy pink. An alarm went off in my head. This color is indicative of a stomach problem. Was the problem really in Peggy's teeth?

My suspicions were confirmed when Peggy told me that, yes, her digestion "was not the best." Furthermore, the tooth she complained about looked healthy to me.

When I took a digital x-ray—enlarged and colorized for better viewing of the tooth nerve—all I saw was healthy tissue. I then performed some kinesiology tests on her of the kind I will describe below.

The result of this test indicated to me that there was an imbalance somewhere in Peggy's body, although at this point I could not exactly pinpoint where.

By now I'd become pretty well convinced that the problem was not the tooth itself. It was a healthy tooth that was just giving off symptoms, so there was no reason to do anything to it.

Just to be certain that the x-rays didn't miss anything, I gave Peggy some homeopathic remedies including Arnica and Hypericum—natural substances derived from plants that help to relieve pain and stress and promote healing.

I also treated Peggy with a tincture of Rescue Remedy, a Bach Flower Remedy. These so-called "flower remedies" were developed years ago by Dr. Edward Bach, a pioneer of flower remedies, who believed that leaf, twig, or flower essences can on a subtle level promote healing in the body.

In addition, I taped a tiny magnet to Peggy's cheek with its north side facing the tooth in order to slow down the growth of harmful bacteria. Magnets have many healing properties, as you will soon see.

After a few days Peggy reported that she was still feeling the throbbing tooth. A few days more passed, and now the young woman said she was experiencing pain in *both* of her lower molars. Again I examined her teeth, and again, all her teeth looked healthy to me.

The two teeth which were bothering Peggy followed one of the meridians, or energy channels, described in Oriental medicine. Because my patient had already mentioned that she suffered from digestive problems, I decided to refer Peggy to an acupuncturist who would work on that meridian.

I was now convinced that Peggy's stomach was signaling for help via the pain in her two molars. The acupuncturist went to work on my patient and her digestion began to improve. Best of all, the pain in her teeth disappeared almost immediately.

Peggy's case is a classic example of why each part of the body must be treated as an integral part of the whole person. It also shows how the holistic dentist who takes a whole-body approach differs significantly from his more mainstream counterpart.

Certainly I am aware that some dental problems require conventional treatment, but never without looking at the whole picture.

Healthy Mouth, Healthy Body

The stories I could tell about connections between oral symptoms and problems in the body such as Peggy experienced are endless. You'd have to be blind not to see how the body functions as a complex whole.

The mouth, as the initial point of entry to the digestive system, can give a dentist like myself a wealth of understanding about a patient's general state of health. That's why holistic dentists use the mouth as a diagnostic area for the entire body.

After years of practicing medicine, I am still surprised at how accurate the mouth can be as an indicator of the body's health, as was the case with Peggy.

The color, shape, and texture of the tongue, gums, and teeth can give the practitioner many clues to a patient's overall health.

Assessing the tongue dates back to 300 B.C., where it was first mentioned in the *Huang Di Nei Jing,* one of the classic texts of Oriental medicine.

The tongue can be considered the body's barometer. If the tongue is pink and has a good texture, the body is usually in a good state of health. If the color is off, such as green, gray, or white, there is usually a problem.

While the scope of this book does not permit me to detail all the alternative healing methods I practice, I do want to introduce you to the disciplines—particularly magnetic therapy, kinesiology, and homeopathy—that I use frequently in my practice. We've touched upon these techniques throughout this book, but I'd like to expand on them right now.

Before I do so, I'd like to introduce you to two dentist friends of mine who have some interesting things to say about alternative healing and stress.

Dr. Robert Veligdan is an assistant professor of dentistry at Columbia University. Bob has been practicing medicine for more than twenty-five years, and was one of the pioneers of porcelain and bonding veneers in the early 1980s. He and I are very much in agreement in our practice of holistic dentistry.

Another friend, Dr. Alan A. Winter, taught clinical periodontics at the postdoctoral level for eleven years, before going on to teach at New York University. He has been in practice for twenty-six years, and has explored the link between stress and dental problems.

V.Z. Bob, what is your approach to holistic dentistry?

R.V. My approach is very much governed by the general rule of dentistry and all medicine: *First, do no harm.* If a treatment may help and does no harm, it is often worth trying.

V.Z. How do you think we holistic dentists are viewed by our patients?

R.V. Practitioners of holistic and alternative medicine are sometimes grouped at health fairs with astrologers, psychics, and such, reflecting their association in some people's minds with things that rely on belief and are thus unscientific.

V.Z. Alan, you and I may disagree over some nutritional issues, but we do agree on the fundamental holistic viewpoint of treating gums and teeth as part of the whole functioning body.

A.W. That's true. The connections between oral symptoms and body conditions are endless. Over the years I've had the task of telling patients that, based on the evidence of their gums, they had all kinds of problems—from AIDS to cancer.

V.Z. Alan, I know you feel as I do that stress can lead to periodontal disease.

A.W. Yes, I put people on vitamins when they show clinical manifestations of stress. For example, people under stress—in my experience it's often women—sometimes develop little balding patches of cilia (cell hairs) on the upper tongue surface. This is known as "burning tongue" or "burning mouth." Stress robs them of the right mix of vitamins. They may not have the right mix of vitamins, such as the B vitamin niacin, and minerals, such as magnesium.

V.Z. Bob, do you believe we can use our life force to heal?

R.V. All the Eastern disciplines make use of the major life force of the body, as utilized, for example, in the twelve meridians of acupuncture and hundreds of acupuncture points. Whether this is "electromagnetic energy" in the Western scientific sense or some kind of "qi energy" is open to debate. The main point is that we *can* use this energy to heal people. We may not know what this energy is or how it works, but we know that it works.

V.Z. Alan, have you ever had any personal experience of herbs working to heal any of your patients?

A.W. One patient comes to mind, a man who had severe periodontal disease and was not responding well to treatment. He told me he was going to use a home remedy for it. At home, he made a preparation of goldenseal and cayenne pepper and rubbed it into his gums. The pain was terrible, he said. But when I next saw him, I observed that his gums were in much better condition.

V.Z. Bob, what about patients who don't buy into all these various energy therapies?

R.V. The patient who benefits doesn't have to believe this is possible. With TMJ problems, for instance, the laying on of hands can transfer some of this life force energy in a healing way. With a TMJ or muscle spasm problem, I put my hand on that side of the face and let the person feel the energy. Sometimes the patient understands what I'm doing, sometimes not. I just do it as a matter of course.

V.Z. Is energy healing just a placebo?

R.V. The mind can play a role in curing. How does the mind do this? In what ways do our expectations work on our bodies? We don't know how—but we know that they do.

Magnet Therapy

Magnetics is an understanding of the interrelationship between the electromagnetic field and the human body, and knowing how to use this relationship to encourage the body to heal itself.

Reported benefits include relief from discomfort, reduction of swelling, and even increased energy. I use magnets in my practice for two things—accelerated healing and the stimulation of organs and all forms of life, including beneficial bacteria.

For those of you who are nonbelievers, I'd suggest taking a magnet and putting it underneath your plants with the south side facing up. In fact, take two plants. Put a magnet under one and leave the other one alone.

In a month, I guarantee that you will see a difference in the growth rate of the plants. The plant with the southern pole will grow twice as fast. It's a very simple experiment, so try it!

The ordinary horseshoe magnet is not used for healing, because the positive and negative poles are too close together. A small light-weight bar magnet is best, because it is easily taped to the body part in need of therapy.

You need to determine which is the north pole and which is the south, because their therapeutic effects are different. Although the magnet you get will probably have N at one end and S at the other, don't assume that N is the north pole and S is the south pole.

Some manufacturers use N to label the north-seeking pole (that is, the south pole) and S to label the south-seeking (north) pole. Because the therapeutic effects of each pole are different, you need to make sure which pole is which on your magnet.

A simple way to verify this is to tie a thread around the center of the magnet and suspend it so that it balances horizontally. The magnet's south pole will point to the geographic north at your location. If you are not sure which way is north, use a compass.

Magnets can be very powerful, but the ones that holistic dentists use for oral therapy don't overpower the body's energy fields. If you are using magnets at home for healing, remember, they are not toys.

Magnets are powerful instruments and you should not start placing them on your body without first becoming familiar with how magnets work.

I use a bar magnet an inch to two inches long that can be conveniently placed in various locations by being taped to the skin. In a moment I'll explain how that works.

HEALING WITH THE MAGNETIC POLES

North pole energy has an arresting effect on bacteria and growths. It controls inflammatory conditions in joints that have redness, warmth, and swelling. North pole energy also has a sedating effect on the nerve tissue, and sedates or inhibits pain.

This side of the magnet can slow down overactive organs, and even reduce acidity by reducing the hydrogen iron and causing alkalinity. All of this will help bring inflamed tissue back to a normal state.

The south pole is positive energy. It helps to stimulate all life forms—including bacteria—so it should *never* be used where there is an infection. South pole energy increases acidity, and is most often used to stimulate underactive glands such as the adrenal, thyroid, and pancreas.

IF YOU'RE USING A MAGNET AT HOME

- Never drop or throw a magnet or strike it sharply.
- Don't break a magnet or chip pieces off.
- Never store a magnet in a very hot place. A magnet can lose its strength at 400 degrees Fahrenheit.
- Do make a "keeper" to close the circuit and retain the energy. Simply bend a piece of steel, iron, or tin into a C shape, so that it makes tight contact with both poles of your magnet.

Therapeutic Effect of Magnets

Some of the earliest experiments on the effect of magnets on living systems were done on plants. Seeds placed under south pole energy for various periods from 6 to 200 hours were planted and grew into hardier, healthier plants than usual. (In the case of vegetable seeds, the yield of the mature plant was greater.)

Meanwhile, seeds placed under north pole energy for similar periods and planted grew into tall, thin plants. The mature vegetables from these seeds had a reduced yield.

Seeds not placed under magnetic energy were planted and grown as controls.

In Florida, Albert Roy Davis and Walter C. Rawls, Jr., authors of *The Magnetic Effect,* found that the proteins, sugars, and oils were higher in vegetables treated as seeds with the south pole of a magnet than those in the control plants.

Vegetables treated as seeds with the north pole were lower in proteins, sugars, and oils than were the control vegetables. Davis and Rawls also increased the sugar production of sugar beets by south pole exposure of seeds. Similar treatment of peanut seeds enhanced the natural peanut oil and protein contents of the mature plants.

Of most interest to us dentists are Davis and Rawls's findings that the north pole energy of a magnet can discourage the growth of bacteria. The north pole energy doesn't kill the bacteria or clear up a bacterial infection, but in many cases, it stops bacterial growth by helping to alkalize the blood in the area.

This gives the body's own defense systems a chance to overcome the invaders. Combining the growth-arresting power of a magnet with an alkalizing diet gives the body an even greater opportunity to restore chemical balance and good health.

Earlier, I mentioned how an infected tooth can be treated by taping a small but powerful magnet to the cheek, so that its north pole is over the area of infection. The energy from the north pole slows down bacterial growth in the infection.

Needless to say, since the magnet's south pole *promotes* growth, you need to be careful not to place that pole over an infection. It's also worth repeating that magnetic energy won't *cure* an infection, but can simply slow it down, giving the body a chance to do its own healing.

By changing the environment in which harmful oral microorganisms like to live, north pole energy can produce positive results with everything from decaying teeth, gum infections, and infected tooth roots, to loose teeth.

I find that patients with loose teeth have a lot of bone loss, with flaccid gum tissue and poor tone. With the mouth rinse, vitamins, minerals, and herbs, we can get that tone back. This, in itself, will help to tighten up the teeth.

I will then have the patient tape the north pole of the magnet over the infected area for 30 to 40 minutes twice a day, in the morning and evening. Using this method, I have seen good results in the healing of the tissue.

For more advanced infections, it may be desirable to apply the magnet for longer periods. After three or four applications, you should notice not only a lessening of discomfort or pain if there is any, but a further tightening up of loose teeth. These magnetic applications must be done over the course of several weeks before any improvement is noticed.

So far, we have only looked at the growth-inhibiting power of north pole energy. Growth-promoting south pole energy aids in tissue healing, but this benefit is offset by the likelihood that bacterial infection will also be promoted at the same time.

Bone growth is sometimes promoted by taping the south pole of a magnet above the problem area and taping the north pole of another magnet below the infected area.

Ileana's Story

Ileana was a twenty-two-year-old member of a classical ballet company. She was lithe and graceful, and had muscle tone that few people manage to achieve. Like all professional dancers, she was used to injury.

She usually coped with injury by denial, saying that she just "worked through it." In one fall, she cracked a tooth and left it untreated. By the time her ballet company arrived in New York for a six-week season, an infection had developed in the gum next to the fracture.

Ileana hadn't seen a dentist since her last year of high school, and other parts of her mouth were showing early signs of gingivitis. Otherwise her health seemed to be excellent.

I expected to encounter no unusual problems in restoring the fractured tooth. But over the course of three weekly visits, I noticed that the infection was persisting in spite of treatment. Ileana was against taking antibiotics except as a last resort.

By that time I had learned what a stressful life she led. Perfection was demanded with every performance, rivalry was encouraged among the dancers, and the company spent long stretches on the road.

The fact that she had not been able to ignore her tooth injury had added to this stress. The stress, in turn, had probably impaired her immune system's healing abilities, and this may have caused the early signs of gingivitis.

I showed Ileana how to tape the north pole of a magnet on her cheek over the infection. I had her promise to wear it for an hour each morning before exercising and each night after performing. In several days, without any antibiotics or other treatments, the infection began to subside.

The day before the company left town, she came by for a final checkup. Her gum infection had completely cleared. My belief is that the north pole energy slowed the infection enough for her immune system to regain control.

The Body's Healing Energy

Some people believe that magnetic therapy works by energizing acupuncture points. According to Oriental medicine, these points occur along twelve acupuncture meridians, or channels, through which the body's *qi*, or healing energy, passes.

A traditional Chinese tale traces the origin of acupuncture back to a warrior who was plagued with ailments for many years. In a battle, he received a shallow spear wound. When the wound healed, he found he had been cured of his chronic ailments.

Presumably the spear pierced an acupuncture point, a point or area along one of the twelve meridians in which an energy blockage had occurred. Since then, it has been learned that by stimulating an acupuncture point, one can get the energy moving again.

According to Chinese medical theory, each meridian is associated with particular organs. It is believed that every two hours, the main body energy passes through one of these different meridians.

The result is that particular organs vary in their vulnerability or strength according to the time of day or night. The following chart indicates the different organs of the body and the times when they are most strongly affected by qi energy.

Meridians and Time Sensitivities

Time	Meridian
1–3 A.M.	Liver
3–5 A.M.	Lung
5–7 A.M.	Large intestine
7–9 A.M.	Stomach
9–11 A.M.	Spleen

11 A.M.–1 P.M.	Heart
1–3 P.M.	Small intestine
3–5 P.M.	Bladder
5–7 P.M.	Kidney
7–9 P.M.	Pericardium
9–11 P.M.	Triple warmer
11 P.M.–1 A.M.	Gallbladder

Oriental Meridians, Teeth, and Body Organs

According to Oriental medicine, the teeth are linked to various organs in the body as follows:

Teeth	Organs
Central and lateral incisors	Kidney, bladder, urinogenital system, rectum
Canines	Eyes, liver, gallbladder
Premolars	Nose, shoulder, elbow, hand, big toe, lung, intestines
First and second molars	Tongue, jaw, ankle bone, pancreas, esophagus
Third molars	Tongue, shoulder, elbow, foot, heart, duodenum, central nervous system

This, of course, is a much-oversimplified overview of a very complex study of the relationship of teeth to the body's organs.

Based on this system, holistic dentists such as myself believe that an infected tooth can cause an energy blockage on an acupuncture meridian and vice versa. While I have seen no hard evidence to support this claim, I nonetheless pay very serious attention to tooth-organ linkages along these channels.

In my practice, it's not unusual to hear a patient complaining about a pain somewhere in the body, only for me to discover a problem with a tooth on the same meridian. After the tooth problem has been treated, the body symptom often disappears.

Small Intestine Meridian

The temporomandibular joint (TMJ)—the upper and lower jaw muscles in front of each ear—are located on a meridian channel linked to the small intestine meridian, according to Oriental medicine.

The channel actually begins at the side of the little finger and continues up the outer edge of the hand, forearm, and elbow. It then moves its energy to the back of the upper arm, the shoulder joint, and across to the scapula.

The meridian then crosses back and forth over the upper trapezius muscle, continues to the back of the neck, and onward toward the cheek. It ends in front of the ear, where the TMJ muscles are located.

If there is an energy blockage anywhere along this small intestine meridian—especially between the hours of 1 and 3 in the afternoon—the following problems can theoretically develop:

Crohn's disease
Digestive problems, intestinal flu, diarrhea
Ear problems, tinnitus, sore throat
Gastric pain
Poor absorption of nutrients
Shoulder or arm pain
Sore TMJ

This connection between the muscles in the jaw and other parts of the body is something that holistic dentists and physicians keep in mind when treating a patient. I have, for example, recommended acupuncture to patients when I could find no dental problem to account for their TMJ symptoms, but suspected an energy problem along that meridian. Since acupuncture by an expert won't harm and may indeed provide relief, the patient has nothing to lose and everything to gain.

Clinical Kinesiology

Clinical kinesiology is a diagnostic system of muscle tests that can detect energy imbalances or dysfunctions in the body before any physical symptoms appear.

This procedure involves having a patient hold the left arm straight out to the side in order for me to test the muscle response. I then place my fingers just above the bridge of the nose.

This is an "energy point," where the life force can be tapped into for diagnostic purposes. With my other hand, I press down on the patient's left wrist.

From that response, I can determine the strength or weakness of the response, and can make deductions about the patient's health.

If, for example, my patient is complaining about a sore tooth, yet I can't find a cause after x-rays and other tests, I'll have the patient touch various places on the body as, each time, I press down on the left arm. When the left arm *does* go weak, the corollary place that was touched can now be investigated as the possible source of the pain.

Clinical kinesiology is a system that was developed in the 1960s by Dr. George Goodheart, who used tests of simple body movements, especially muscle movements, to evaluate the body's level of physical functioning. More than fifty-four muscle tests were used.

His colleague, Dr. Alan Beardall, developed this system even further. By the mid-1970s, Dr. Beardall had developed more than 250 muscle tests that focused primarily on muscle reflexes.

This new diagnostic method became known as *clinical kinesiology,* and is practiced by many holistic doctors and dentists today.

I became involved with kinesiology testing quite by accident. I had a patient about twenty-five years ago, when I first started doing holistic work, who had missing teeth, and I needed to put crowns in. When I did that, I changed her bite a little bit, and that affected her jaw muscles, or TMJs.

She called up to tell me a most remarkable story. It turned out that she had been having trouble walking down stairs. Her balance was off, and she had been treated by various doctors for over a year. Nothing had shown up.

The minute I changed that bite, it somehow affected the muscle in her jaw and her sense of balance suddenly and mysteriously returned. I became very interested in the whole field of muscle testing, which eventually led me to study kinesiology.

It's interesting to me to compare acupuncture with clinical kinesiology. In acupuncture, each acupuncture point contains energy potential. When stimulated, an acupuncture point can help the body energy move along a meridian.

Clinical kinesiology is more of a diagnostic system—an investigative tool—than a means of unblocking energy. Each cell, body part, organ, and energy system can be seen as being genetically encoded to work for the survival of the organism.

The brain acts like a telephone switching center or computer to channel body energy to maintain body function and to process, store, and retrieve information. As connections are made, body energy flows. Muscle tests tap into this network and reveal information I'd be unable to obtain otherwise.

A Kinesiology Tryout

What I typically do to determine if there is, for example, a TMJ problem is to have my patient hold the left hand parallel to the floor, with teeth gently pressed together. I then press down on the arm and observe the normal resistance strength.

Next, I repeat this muscle-testing motion with the patient's mouth open. Then, I switch to the other side of the body and repeat the tests. If the jaw is not aligned properly, the arm resistance on either one or both sides will be weaker when the mouth is open.

After I determine where the problem is, I will manipulate my patient's facial bones and muscles with my fingers to produce relief and restore the jawbones to a proper working relationship. I then find out what caused the problem in the first place, and work with the patient toward making certain it does not return.

Before we move on to the next chapter and a discussion of another alternative healing method I often use—homeopathy—let me say here that I believe dentists of the future will routinely use procedures such as kinesiology, magnetic therapy, and other such modalities as part of their routine screenings.

The influence of Oriental medicine is growing at an incredible rate, and so are many other alternative healing techniques. Today, more and more hospitals are utilizing everything from hands-on healing to reiki and reflexology.

Dentistry will not be far behind!

CHAPTER 20

Homeopathic Healers

For more than 200 years, homeopathic medicine has been used to stimulate the body's natural ability to heal itself. These "medicines" are created from naturally derived substances from gold to snake venom.

In fact, until the wonder drug penicillin was discovered, homeopathic remedies were used by physicians as natural antibiotics for dozens of diseases. They were first introduced in the 1700s, when Dr. Samuel Hahnemann, who was also a chemist, mineralogist, and botanist, first formulated them.

Homeopathy is closely related to the use of vaccines, where minuscule amounts of highly refined extracts of disease-causing agents are used to prevent the diseases they would normally cause.

The homeopathic dental remedies I use are almost like natural vaccines, and they work on the principle that "like cures like." These remedies—consisting of herbs, nutrients, and other natural substances—are administered in small amounts to get the immune system working. The same substances that can induce symptoms in a healthy person are used to cure those symptoms in someone who is sick.

A state of healthy physiological balance is known as homeostasis.

When one system goes out of balance and threatens sickness, your body tries to adjust to this disturbance and restore homeostasis.

As long as your body chemistry and functions stay in balance or are restored quickly to balance, you will stay healthy. When that doesn't happen, homeopathic remedies can help encourage the body to do so.

All the homeopathic remedies I use are directed at arousing and strengthening a person's own natural healing process. In the final result, it is you, the patient, who must heal himself or herself.

When treating patients, homeopathic practitioners—including us dentists—always keep homeostasis in mind. We try to find out what caused a body's chemical balance to get out of kilter in the first place, and then search for ways to restore the body to homeostasis.

I have used many homeopathic remedies over the years, for everything from reducing swelling and discomfort in postoperative patients, to helping patients feel less stress and anxiety. I use homeopathic remedies because, as a whole body doctor, I prefer them over antibiotics and prescription pain killers.

And I have not yet been disappointed by the results that I've achieved from this natural alternative to the antibiotics that drug companies turn out at high cost.

Of course, I don't just rely on homeopathic remedies. There are times when I feel that an antibiotic or a painkiller is more to the point, and I will certainly prescribe that.

I have had patients come into my office with such pain in their mouths, that they were literally begging for instant relief. Homeopathy is not a quick-acting cure, so in such a case a painkiller is in order.

For less critical situations, however, I will certainly suggest to them that they give homeopathy a try.

NINE MUSTS OF HOMEOPATHIC MEDICINE

The following nine requirements should be met by all health professionals before they practice homeopathic medicine.

1. Their attempts to restore patient health should be immediate, nontraumatic, and lasting in effect.

2. They must never use remedies that cause side effects.
3. They must clearly distinguish between health and disease.
4. They must determine whether a patient's disease can be alleviated or cured.
5. They must become familiar with the homeopathic remedies appropriate for the most frequently seen ailments.
6. They must know the most likely physical reaction to each remedy they employ.
7. They must be able to recognize immediately any side effect or unusual reaction to a remedy.
8. They must be able to tell when an apparent worsening of a patient's symptoms is actually a sign of healing.
9. They must be able to tell what to recommend a remedy for, what dose to give, how long the dose will last, when to repeat the dose, when to stop it, and when to change to another remedy.

How I Use Homeopathy

Bleeding gums, sores, and neuralgia or facial pain are all conditions that can be helped by homeopathic medicine.

I suggest either single substances—such as Ferrum phosphoricum, for bleeding—or a combination of remedies for slow absorption under the tongue. I also suggest homeopathic combinations for toothaches, dental infections, TMJ problems, and much more.

Some homeopathic medicines that I prescribe are for postoperative oral pain and discomfort. These remedies will act both as tranquilizer and an aid to tissue healing. Arnica, for example, is excellent for stress, and Coffea cruda works well as a tranquilizer. If a patient is really panicked, I might suggest Aconite.

I also used an oral detox combination that can help fight off the effects of mercury poisoning from amalgam fillings. If a patient has lots of allergies and is really sick, I will prescribe what is called a "lymph drainage combination."

This consists of extracts such as lymph, mammary, spleen, and thymus. There would also be some citrus, echinacea, and other substances added to it. I've used this many times and it's been very successful for patients who have had allergies, and viral colds.

If I find mouth ulcers—especially on the tongue—I might recommend Ars,alb. 30c or Kalibich. 30c for their treatment. All of these remedies are widely used and are found in most—if not all—health food stores and many pharmacies.

In my own home I always keep a homeopathic remedy called Arnica around. It's one of the best remedies I know of for bruising. When my kids were small and fell down and bruised themselves, I'd give them some Arnica and the bruises would go away within a day. The kids have grown up, but I still keep Arnica in the medicine chest.

Remedy Types and Strengths

Homeopathic medicines are available as pellets, tablets, and liquids. Creams and salves can also be used to relieve sore muscles, such as in the face and neck when you have a TMJ problem.

You can make a cream or salve by mixing a remedy in liquid form with a cream or gel base. Pellets and tablets have a milk sugar base. They should be dissolved under the tongue, without chewing. Liquid remedies are dissolved in alcohol and usually taken with an eyedropper.

The potency of a homeopathic remedy is usually indicated by a number followed by the letter X. In this homeopathic decimal system, the number represents the number of zeroes of dilution. For example, 2X signifies a dilution of 1:100, and 3X a dilution of 1:1,000.

Less commonly, the C or centissimal system is used. Here the number before C represents half the zeroes of dilution. For example, 2C signifies a dilution of 1:10,000, and 3C a dilution of 1:1,000,000. The most common strength prescribed is 30C.

HOW MUCH? HOW OFTEN?

General rules of thumb for various potencies and how to use them are given below. All these potencies are available already mixed in small bottles or in tablets and pellets at most health food stores. Always read the labels for a more exact dosage of each product.

- Low-potency remedies (under 12X): For first aid, every 5 to 30 minutes. For an acute condition, every 30 to 60 minutes, decreasing to three to four times a day.
- Medium-potency remedies (12X to 30X): One to three times a day.
- High-potency remedies (30X to 200X): Once a day.

Dental Homeopathic Prescriptions

The homeopathic medicines that are listed here should be used as a general guide. Consult a homeopath for individualized advice. You should also consult your physician before giving homeopathic remedies to children or taking them while pregnant or breastfeeding.

The range of sources for these prescriptions is vast. It includes plant materials, minerals, extracts of chemical compounds, bacterial products, root parts, seeds, and salts such as sodium chloride.

Today, there are more than 2500 substances that have been prepared as homeopathic medicines, and the following list is mainly geared toward dental problems.

While taking homeopathic remedies, don't consume caffeine in any form, raw garlic, or any kind of mint flavoring. Also, avoid breathing in chlorine or eucalyptus. These inactivate the effect of the remedy.

Uses of Homeopathic Remedies

For all of the following, it is best to consult a homeopathic practitioner before use. However, in an emergency, you can safely use 4 pills at a 30C dosage every 3 hours, until the symptoms disappear. If symptoms persist after 2 days on the remedy, seek other help.

You'll find that, with the assistance of a skilled homeopathic practitioner, the following remedies can go a long way towards achieving a healthy mouth in a healthy body.

Abscess

Belladonna	Relieves redness and throbbing.
Bryonia	When pain is relieved by pressure.
Hepar sulphuris	When pus is present.
Myristica	For swelling and numbness.
Pulsatilla	Eases pain.
Pyrogenium	When pus is present but not draining.
Silicea	Speeds the draining of pus.

Bleeding

Arnica	With sore bruising.
Ferrum phosphoricum	Bright red bleeding.
Phosphorus	Persistent bleeding.

Cold Sores

Calcarea carbonica

Discomfort after Treatment

Apis mellifica	Postinjection soreness.
Chamomilla	When taken before visit, increases tolerance of pain.
Hypericum	Nerve injury.
Ledum	Postinjection soreness.
Magnesia phosporica	Jaw stiffness or soreness.
Staphysagria	Heals gum tissue.
Symphytum	Helps bone tissue.

Gum Disease

Arsenicum album	Bleeding gums.
China	Bleeding gums.
Ferrum phosphoricum	Bright red bleeding.

Hepar sulphuris	Suppuration and chronic abscesses.
Hypericum	Tender gums.
Kali chloricum	Ulcerative tissue.
Mercurius solubilis	Ulcerative tissue with coated tongue and metallic taste.
Naturium muriaticum	Strengthens gums.
Nux vomica	Swollen, painful gums with whitish coating of tongue.
Phosphorus	For swollen gums that easily bleed or for too much saliva.
Ruta graveolens	Cavitation and osteonecrosis.
Silicea	For gum abscesses with swollen glands.
Staphysagria	Loose teeth and pressure pain.
Symphytum	Helps ulcerative gums heal.

Neuralgia

Aconite	Trigeminal neuralgia.
Aranea diadema	For radiating pain on right side of face made worse by cold or for sudden tooth pain before sleep.
Cuprum metallicum	Facial muscle cramps.
Gelsemium sempervirens	For headache and neck and upper back pain or for dizziness or numbness.
Ignacia	Piercing headache.
Lachesis	Problems on left side of mouth.
Lycopodium	Problems on right side of mouth.
Magnesia phosphorus	Spasmodic pain worsened by cold and eased by heat and rubbing.
Sanguinaria	Neuralgia and migraine on right side of face.
Spigella	Pain in eye, cheek, and left temple.

Zincum phosphoricum	Sharp pain on right side of head.
Zincum valerian	Sharp pain on left side of head.

Salivation

Baryta carbonica	Excessive salivation during sleep.
Bryonia alba	Dry mouth with great thirst.
Phosphorus	For excessive salivation or for swollen and bleeding gums.
Pulsatilla	Diminished salivation with no thirst.

Stress

Aconite	Restlessness, fright, or panic attacks.
Calcarea carbonica	Fear, weariness, hopelessness, or worries at end of day.
Coffea cruda	Tranquilizer.
Chamomilla	Tranquilizer, sleep promoter, aid to withstanding pain.
Nux vomica	For irritable or nervous people with gastric problems.
Pulsatilla	Anxiety.

Teeth Grinding

Belladonna	Pain.
Podophyllum	Burning tongue sensation.
Tuberculinum	Childhood grinding.

Temporomandibular Joint (TMJ)

Arum triphyllum	Joint pain on swallowing.
Calcarea fluorica	Overly movable joints.
Calcarea phosphorica	Jaws locked shut.
Carbo vegetabilis	Vertigo with nausea and tinnitus.

Chamomilla	For spasms of pain radiating to the ear or for those with low pain tolerance.
Cuprum metallicum	Jaw muscle spasms.
Granatum	Painful cracking of joints.
Magnesium phosphorica	Muscle spasms.
Phytolacca decanda	Ear aches with teeth, jaw, and throat pain.
Rhus toxicodendron	Joint stiffness that is relieved by movement and TMJ popping.

Toothache

Antimonium crudum	Toothache that worsens at night and is made worse by heat.
Aranea diadema	Sudden tooth pain before sleep.
Belladonna	Throbbing pain worsened by pressure.
Calcarea carbonica	Pain worsened by hot or cold air.
Chamomilla	Pain worsened by heat and not eased by cold.
Coffea cruda	Pain worsened by heat but eased by ice.
Ferrum metallicum	Pain eased by ice water.
Magnesia carbonica	Pain worse at night but eased by walking.
Magnesia phosphorica	Pain worsened by cold and eased by heat.
Plantago major	Pain worsened by cold air but eased by pressure.
Pulsatilla	Pain eased by cold water.
Staphysagria	Pain from extensive tooth decay.

Ulcers

Nitricum acidum

CHAPTER 21

The Pick of the Crop

For too long we've tended to look at herbs as an exotic form of alternative healing. We have taken a similar view of homeopathy, magnets, and other such modalities.

I'm glad to say that such attitudes are gradually changing. The use of herbs, for example, is gaining more and more acceptance—not only in the medical profession—but in the world of dentistry as well. Of late, I've seen more herbal products advertised in dental catalogs than ever before—and that's a good start.

There are literally hundreds of herbs that can be used for healing—many of them for a variety of oral problems. While there are way too many to list, in this chapter I've selected my favorites—the pick of the crop.

There are various ways to take herbs—from infusions to decoctions and extracts. Basically, an *infusion* is a herbal tea made by boiling herbs in water. You usually pour a pint of boiling water over a half-ounce to an ounce of plants.

Some preparations require boiling the plants and water together. The plants usually steep for 10 minutes in a glass, ceramic, or enamel pot, with a cover to prevent evaporation.

Strain the tea into a glass or mug. Sip or take spoonfuls of herbal tea over a period of time. Depending on the herb and your ailment, 1 to 4 cups daily may be recommended. Don't drink more than is recommended, and don't drink large amounts in a hurry.

A *decoction* results from boiling plants in water to extract their active ingredients. Roots, seeds, and bark are the parts that are usually boiled. Generally, you will use about an ounce of plant materials to 1 cup of water, which is boiled for 3 to 4 minutes. Then you allow the water to steep from 2 to 10 minutes. Strain out the plant parts before drinking or otherwise using the decoction.

Extracts are the most effective way to take herbs. They are made by pressing the herbs with a hydraulic press and soaking them in water or alcohol for 8 to 12 hours.

An *extract* of an herb is obtained by steeping it in cold water in a nonmetallic or enamel pot for 8 to 12 hours. You then strain the plants from the extract before you drink or use it.

You can juice herbs by chopping them into small pieces and pressing them to squeeze out the juice. Add a little water to the chopped pieces and press for a second time to squeeze out additional juice.

A herb *juice* contains water-soluble vitamins and nutrients and preserves nutrients destroyed by heat. Because these nutrients tend to break down quickly, you should drink the herb juice without delay.

To make a *powder* out of herbs, use a mortar and pestle to grind up dried herbs until you have a fine powder. You can add the powder to water, beverages, or soup, sprinkle it over food, or put it in gelatin capsules. The usual dose for a herbal powder is the amount you can pick up on the tip of a dinner knife.

Herbs can also come in *tincture* form. A herbal tincture is composed of active ingredients of the plant preserved in alcohol. These you can buy at most health food stores and at many pharmacies. Some tinctures also come in water, if you prefer not to take alcohol into your system.

Obtaining Herbs

Depending on where you live, you can find herbs in the wild. Proper identification of plants is vital. You will need the assistance of someone experienced before you get the hang of this, unless you have a well-illustrated field guide. Never use a plant unless you are positive about its identity. Any doubt, throw it out! It may be poisonous.

You can also grow herbs from seeds in your garden or in flowerpots on a balcony or windowsill. However, some herbalists claim that cultivated plants are less effective in healing than wild ones.

When you obtain herbs in the wild or grow your own, you need to dry them for future use. Place them on a clean sheet of paper or shelf or hang them in a dry, well-ventilated place, out of direct sunlight.

Large roots, bulbs, and pieces of bark need to be cut into smaller pieces to dry well. When the plant parts are completely dried, store them in jars made of dark glass that have airtight lids. Light and oxygen cause them to lose potency. Keep the jars in a cool, dry place. Because of the gradual loss of potency, don't store dried herbs for more than a year.

Most people, as we have said, can get their herbs in pill, powder, or tincture form at their local health food store or pharmacy. There are a number of advantages to this, chief of which are convenience and reliable dosage information.

Dosage

There is no exact science about how much of a particular herb you should take, only general guidelines.

Buying commercially prepared pills, capsules, powders, or tinctures makes understanding dosages much easier. Before using a commercial herbal product, read the label and follow its instructions carefully.

If the product doesn't have clear instructions, don't purchase it. Remember: Taking more of a herb does not mean getting additional benefits. Herbs don't work this way. The amount recommended is the one that delivers the maximum benefit.

The Pick of the Crop

Aloe Vera

A perennial that grows in the Southern states, aloe vera has tough, fleshy, spear-like leaves. It's best known for the power of the gel in its leaves to heal and soothe burns. But this herb also has an array of other therapeutic properties.

The gel is also effective for skin problems and is an ingredient in many commercial cosmetics and dermatological products. Aloe is known to be antibacterial, antifungal, and antiviral. It seems to be effective against cold sores.

This herb enhances T-cell function and interferon production in the immune system, and also has antiallergenic and antiinflammatory powers. Its ability to heal gum tissue makes it a valuable ingredient of many mouth rinses.

Many people keep an aloe plant and apply gel directly to their skin from broken open leaves. Both skin and oral preparations are available. Aloe is not recommended for deep, open wounds, because it may slow healing.

Astragalus

The legume astragalus is a primary herb in Chinese traditional medicine, used to restore weakened *qi* (body energy). To help relieve a painful outbreak of cold sores, take equal amounts of the following herbs: astragalus, yellow dock, red sage, myrrh, echinacea, and marshmallow. Boil in water for 5 minutes and then steep for another 10 minutes. Apply the liquid to the affected area with cotton swabs.

Bee Propolis

Propolis is the brownish resinous material collected by bees from tree buds and utilized as a cement. It has antibacterial properties. To ease a toothache, mix powdered turmeric, chamomile, and echinacea with a little water and bee propolis until you have a muddy solution. Apply this to the tooth for as long as necessary.

Black Walnut

Black walnut is a forest tree that grows in the temperate zone of eastern North America. To jump-start healing from tooth pain, try a combination of cayenne pepper, echinacea, goldenseal root, myrrh gum, yarrow, marshmallow root, black walnut hulls, and turmeric root. Applying black walnut to cold sores may also help.

Burdock

The root, seeds, and leaves of burdock are used. The plant grows wild in both North America and Europe. A standard infusion is made of crushed seeds, or a strong decoction of the root. A combination of goldenseal, red clover, and burdock can help relieve the discomfort of cold sores.

Some dentists use burdock root, olive leaf extract, and oil of oregano as natural antimicrobial agents in cleaned cavitations to induce healing and filling with new bone.

Calendula

Well known for its healing properties, calendula contains many immune system stimulators, such as flavonoids and carotenoids. It is a garden plant of the marigold type.

Calendula soothes and helps heal tissues.

An excellent homemade herbal mouth rinse can be made from the tinctures of calendula, myrrh, and goldenseal. Mix equal parts in a brown bottle. Always shake well before using. Use 1 teaspoon of herbal tincture in 1 cup of water and place the mixture in a herbal irrigator such as a Water Pik.

Do not take calendula internally while pregnant.

Cayenne Pepper

Also known as chili or red hot pepper, cayenne pepper comes from the fruit of a tropical shrub. Its active ingredient is capsaicin. Cayenne pepper is a powerful antioxidant and helps reduce cholesterol and triglyceride levels. It seems to be effective against cold sores.

Because cayenne pepper diminishes skin pain by depleting sensory nerve fibers of the neurotransmitter substance P, it's often applied to the skin to reduce the pain of trigeminal neuralgia *(tic douloureux)*. This kind of neuralgia can be associated with cavitations and osteonecrosis. The skin salve is likely to be called capsaicin rather than cayenne pepper.

To jump-start healing from tooth pain, try a combination of cayenne pepper, echinacea, goldenseal root, myrrh gum, yarrow, marshmallow root, black walnut hulls, and turmeric root.

Chamomile

Chamomile (also spelled camomile) grows wild in Europe, and is sometimes called Roman chamomile to distinguish it from German chamomile, which resembles it but belongs to a different genus.

Chamomile tea is one of the most popular herbal teas, for its calming properties and as an aid to digestion. To ease a toothache, mix the powdered forms of turmeric, chamomile, and echinacea with a little water and bee propolis until you have a muddy solution.

Apply this to the tooth for as long as necessary. Calendula and chamomile soothe and help heal tissues, while turmeric and echinacea fight infection.

Chaparral

Chaparral is one of the most powerful herbal antibiotics, effective against viruses, bacteria, and parasites. It is also an immune system booster. This herb assists in the recovery from cold sores. In tincture form, 10 to 30 drops should be taken at least three times a day.

Clove Oil

The familiar clove used in cooking is the dried flower bud of the clove tree, which grows in the tropics. Clove oil is one of the most effective painkillers for toothache found in nature.

However, because it can irritate gums, you need to dilute clove oil with an equal amount of olive oil or vegetable oil. Apply this mixture with a cotton swab to the aching tooth. You should find immediate relief from pain, which can last up to an hour. You can use whole cloves for this, but clove oil is more penetrating and effective in killing pain.

Dandelion

This common herb, a relative of chicory, grows wild in temperate climates throughout the world. Although the root is the part most often used, the entire plant has medicinal value. Dandelion leaves make an excellent salad or lightly cooked green vegetable.

Tea can be made from the leaves, organic wine from the flowers, and a coffee substitute from the roots. To help slow the decay process in teeth, try a mixture of chickweed, dandelion, spiderwort, plantain, mugwort, and seaweed.

To help deal with inflammation caused by cold sores, mix 3 drops of each of the following in a half-glass of water: echinacea, white willow bark, St. John's wort, white pine bark, devil's claw root, red clover, gotu kola, alfalfa, dandelion, and ginger. Take this four times a day.

Dandelion is available in many forms. To my knowledge, no toxic reactions or side effects have ever been reported, for either internal or external use.

Devil's Claw

The root of devil's claw contains many active ingredients, a number of which are beneficial for arthritic and rheumatic conditions, as well as for lowering cholesterol levels. Devil's claw is effective for neuralgia pain.

To help deal with inflammation caused by cold sores, mix three drops of each of the following tinctures in a half-glass of water: echinacea, white willow bark, St. John's wort, white pine bark, devil's claw root, red clover, gotu kola, alfalfa, dandelion, and ginger. Take this four times a day.

Because of its bitterness, devil's claw is taken in tablet form. It should not be taken while pregnant.

Echinacea

Echinacea or purple coneflower is a perennial herb that grows throughout middle America. This herb contains at least seven different categories of active ingredients. It's even an effective remedy for snakebite.

Echinacea is used in mouth rinses as an antibacterial agent and because it increases the number of T-cells and plasma cells, enhances antibody production, stimulates the immune system, and neutralizes toxins.

When combined with other herbs, it helps control inflammation. Because it boosts the immune system, echinacea helps suppress cold sores. To help relieve a painful outbreak of cold sores, take equal amounts of the following herbs:

Astragalus, yellow dock, red sage, myrrh, echinacea, and marshmallow. Boil in water for 5 minutes and then steep for another 10 minutes. Apply the liquid to the affected area with cotton swabs.

To help deal with inflammation caused by cold sores, mix 3 drops of each of the following in a half-glass of water: echinacea, white willow bark, St. John's wort, white pine bark, devil's claw root, red clover, gotu kola, alfalfa, dandelion, and ginger. Take this four times a day.

To jump-start healing from tooth pain, try a combination of cayenne pepper, echinacea, goldenseal root, myrrh gum, yarrow, marshmallow root, black walnut hulls, and turmeric root.

Echinacea is safe at recommended doses.

Garlic

A member of the lily family, garlic can be used as a spice or medicinal herb, either fresh or in dried form. Its active ingredient is a volatile oil containing sulfur compounds.

Garlic is a useful ingredient in detox diets and helps prevent tooth decay. When combined with myrrh, it helps prevent tooth pain. In two divided doses per day, 1200 to 2400 milligrams of garlic extract is effective in combating gum disease.

Taken two or three times a day, garlic supplements can help relieve the discomfort of cold sores. Taken with beta-carotenes and a high-multivitamin/mineral supplement, 250 milligrams of garlic four times a day can help an infected tooth.

Two capsules three times a day stimulate the immune system. You can add garlic to any nutrients you are taking to detoxify from amalgam fillings.

I recommend putting garlic in all kinds of foods. However, garlic causes gastrointestinal irritation in some people, and others may be allergic to its sulfur-containing compounds.

German Chamomile

German chamomile (also spelled camomile) is a different herb from chamomile, which it resembles in appearance. For tooth pain, add two dried flowers to a half-cup of boiling water and let cool. Take a mouthful at a time and hold in the mouth for a while.

Also for relief of tooth pain, use mullein as a tincture with balm or German chamomile. Mullein seems to augment the painkilling properties of the others.

Ginger

Jamaica is the biggest exporter of cultivated ginger, which is grown throughout the Tropics. The root is the part used for both cooking and healing. If you use a root, make sure to get an unpeeled one, since the peeled form has lost much of its essential oils.

Ginger oil is steam distilled from fresh roots. Gingerol is thought to be its most active ingredient. A tincture or powdered mixture of ginger and slippery elm relieves tooth pain.

A tea made from ginger, white willow, rosemary, wood betony, heartsease, skullcap, red raspberry, and valerian is an effective reliever of tooth pain.

For cold sores, mix 3 drops of each of the following in a half-glass of water: ginger, echinacea, white willow bark, St. John's wort, white pine bark, devil's claw root, red clover, gotu kola, alfalfa, and dandelion. Take this four times a day.

In addition, ginger is known to have antioxidant and antibiotic powers and lower cholesterol. It functions as a painkiller in much the same way as the capsaicin in cayenne pepper.

There is no agreement about the best way to take ginger or in what amount. Some people suffer gastrointestinal discomfort from eating too much ginger.

Gingko Biloba

Extracts from the leaves of gingko biloba or the maidenhair tree are used medicinally. This ancient tree is a staple of Chinese traditional medicine. Taking 60 milligrams of its supplement in tablet form twice a day supports the central nervous system during mercury detoxification from amalgam fillings.

Ginko acts as an antioxidant in brain cells, scavenging free radicals. Gingko biloba also stabilizes nerve cell membranes and enhances blood supply to the brain.

This herb also increases nerve transmission rate, assists in the synthesis of neurotransmitters, and assists receptors for the neurotransmitter acetylcholine in the hippocampus area of the brain. It has a wide array of other effects in the body.

The strength of dried leaves and crude extracts varies so widely, they are difficult to use. The standardized extract usually recommends a dosage of 40 milligrams three times a day.

Goldenseal

Goldenseal grows wild in the Eastern states and is cultivated in the Northwest. Its dried roots are the parts used for healing. The alkaloid berberine is the most important active ingredient.

Since berberine is also the active ingredient of Oregon grape and some other herbs, their effects are similar to those of goldenseal. To jump-start healing from tooth pain, try a combination of cayenne pepper, echinacea, goldenseal root, myrrh gum, yarrow, marshmallow root, black walnut hulls, and turmeric root.

Goldenseal is used in mouth rinses as an astringent and booster of the immune system. A combination of goldenseal, red clover, and burdock can help relieve the discomfort of cold sores.

Goldenseal is recommended for inflammations of the mucous membranes. A mouth rinse of white oak bark and goldenseal helps take away the pain and swelling caused by toothache.

An excellent homemade herbal mouth rinse can be made from the tinctures of calendula, myrrh, and goldenseal. Mix equal parts in a brown bottle. Always shake well before using. Use 1 teaspoon of herbal tincture in 1 cup of water and place the mixture in a herbal irrigator such as a Water Pik.

Because preparations vary widely in quality, you should choose a standardized extract. Avoid berberine-containing plants when you are pregnant.

Gotu Kola

The entire gotu kola plant is used. Known also as centella, it grows in the Southern hemisphere. Triterpenoid compounds are the active ingredients, not all of which have been identified.

One cup of gotu kola tea daily is widely used to heal tissues and promote tissue growth. To help deal with inflammation caused by cold sores, mix 3 drops (from a tincture) of each of the following in a half-glass of water: echinacea, white willow bark, St. John's wort, white pine bark, devil's claw root, red clover, gotu kola, alfalfa, dandelion, and ginger. Take this four times a day. This herb also helps gums heal from periodontal disease.

Licorice

The major active component of licorice is glycyrrhizin, derived from the root of this temperate zone shrub. However, because of possible side effects (sodium and water retention), deglycyrrhizinated licorice (DGL) is usually used. Its antibacterial action helps reduce tooth decay.

Powdered DGL, mixed with water, applied directly to an aching tooth is highly effective in relieving pain. The antiinflammatory and healing properties of licorice help skin recover quickly from a cold sore.

For cold sores in the mouth, use a mouth rinse four times a day consisting of 200 milligrams of powdered DGL dissolved in 200 milliliters of warm water. DGL is also a well known remedy for gastric and intestinal ulcers.

Licorice in any form should probably not be used by people who have high blood pressure, have suffered renal failure, or take digitalis.

Marshmallow

Marshmallow is a relative of the hollyhock. Its leaves and roots are used by herbalists. To help relieve a painful outbreak of cold sores, take equal amounts of the following herbs: astragalus, yellow dock, red sage, myrrh, echinacea, and marshmallow. Boil in water for 5 minutes then steep for another 10 minutes. Apply the liquid to the affected area with cotton swabs.

Milk Thistle

Milk thistle, also known as Mary thistle, marian thistle, lady's thistle, holy thistle, and wild artichoke, grows in Europe and some parts of America. The active ingredient, silymarin, is most concentrated in the fruit, but occurs also in the leaves and seeds.

You can take 70 to 200 milligrams three times a day in capsule form as part of a detox diet. Milk thistle's beneficial effects are mostly felt by the liver. Silymarin has improved the functions of livers damaged by drugs, chemicals, or alcohol. It combats both acute and chronic viral hepatitis.

Mugwort

Mugwort grows as a weed worldwide. The leaves are used to make tea or a tincture. They can also be smoked. To help slow the decay process in teeth, try a mixture of chickweed, dandelion, spiderwort, plantain, mugwort, and seaweed. Don't take mugwort internally when you are pregnant.

Mullein

Mullein grows wild in the eastern half of the United States. For relief of tooth pain, use mullein as a tincture with balm or German chamomile. Mullein seems to augment the painkilling properties of the others.

Myrrh

The resin is used of the gum myrrh tree, which grows in parts of Africa and the Middle East. An excellent homemade herbal mouth rinse can be made from the tinctures of calendula, myrrh, and goldenseal.

Mix equal parts in a brown bottle. Always shake well before using. Use 1 teaspoon of herbal tincture in 1 cup of water and place the mixture in a herbal irrigator such as a Water Pik.

To help relieve a painful outbreak of cold sores, take equal amounts of the following herbs: astragalus, yellow dock, red sage, myrrh, echinacea, and marshmallow. Boil in water for 5 minutes and then steep for another 10 minutes. Apply the liquid to the affected area with cotton swabs.

Myrrh should not be taken while you are pregnant or if you have kidney trouble.

Olive Leaf

Olive tree leaves can be made into tea to lower high blood pressure or reduce fever or nervous tension. Some dentists use burdock root, olive leaf extract, and oil of oregano as natural antimicrobial agents in cleaned cavitations to induce healing and filling with new bone.

Parsley

Taken as either a food or medicinal herb, parsley contains nutrients that help to combat periodontal disease.

Pennyroyal

Pennyroyal grows as a weed in the eastern half of the United States. Tea made from pennyroyal is effective against tooth pain. Pennyroyal was used in the nineteenth century, with brewers yeast, to induce abortion, and so should not be taken during pregnancy. Its oil should never be taken internally.

Plantain

Plantain grows wild in the eastern half of the United States and along the Pacific coast. Its leaves and seeds have diuretic and antiinflammatory properties.

To help slow the decay process in teeth, try a mixture of chickweed, dandelion, spiderwort, plantain, mugwort, and seaweed. For tooth pain, mix the powder of either plantain root or leaves with water and apply the paste directly to the tooth.

Prickly Ash

Prickly ash is a native tree of eastern North America. The powder of prickly ash bark can be chewed or brushed on the gums to relieve a toothache or treat gum disease.

Rose

The ordinary red garden rose has long been used by herbalists. The parts used are the flowers and hips. Those from red roses are thought to be better than others.

Of the horticultural types of red roses, Hybrid Perpetuals are considered the most suitable. A decoction of red roses and wine is good for toothache. To make, boil the petals for 5 minutes and then steep for another 10. Mix with a small amount of any type of wine and rinse.

Rosemary

Rosemary is a widely cultivated, popular cooking herb, as well as having medicinal properties. A tea made from ginger, white willow bark, rosemary, wood betony, heartsease, skullcap, red raspberry, and valerian is an effective reliever of tooth pain.

St. John's Wort

Long popular as an antidepressant in Germany and other European countries, St. John's wort has become a much publicized remedy in recent years in America. It grows wild in Europe and America, especially in northern California and southern Oregon.

As well as being an antidepressant, it is an antiviral agent. To help deal with inflammation caused by cold sores, mix 3 drops of each of the following in a half-glass of water: echinacea, white willow bark, St. John's wort, white pine bark, devil's claw root, red clover, gotu kola, alfalfa, dandelion, and ginger. Take this four times a day.

Slippery Elm

Also known as red elm, slippery elm is a tree, the inner bark of which has medicinal properties. A tincture or powdered mixture of ginger and slippery elm relieves tooth pain.

Turmeric

Turmeric, a member of the ginger family, is grown in the Asian tropics. Boiled, cleaned, sun-dried, and polished, the root is used for medicinal purposes and as the main ingredient of curry powder. Curcumin and some volatile oils are believed to be its most pharmacologically active agents.

Turmeric is an antioxidant and appears to inhibit steps in the cancer process. It has long been used as an antiinflammatory agent in Ayurvedic medicine.

To ease a toothache, mix the powdered forms of turmeric, chamomile, and echinacea with a little water and bee propolis until you have a muddy solution. Apply this to the tooth for as long as necessary. Calendula and chamomile soothe and help heal tissues, while turmeric and echinacea fight infection.

To jump-start healing from tooth pain, try a combination of cayenne pepper, echinacea, goldenseal root, myrrh gum, yarrow, marshmallow root, black walnut hulls, and turmeric root. At very high doses, turmeric may cause irritation of the gastric or intestinal walls.

White Oak

White oak is a tree native to the eastern half of North America. Its bark is used medicinally. A mouth rinse of white oak bark and goldenseal helps take away the pain and swelling caused by toothache.

White Pine

This large evergreen tree grows in eastern North America. The inner bark and young shoots are used by herbalists. To help deal with inflammation caused by cold sores, mix 3 drops from a tincture of each of the following in a half-glass of water: echinacea, white willow bark, St. John's wort, white pine bark, devil's claw root, red clover, gotu kola, alfalfa, dandelion, and ginger. Take this four times a day.

Yellow Dock

Yellow dock grows as a weed in North America and Europe. To help relieve a painful outbreak of cold sores, take equal amounts of the following herbs: astragalus, yellow dock, red sage, myrrh, echinacea, and marshmallow. Boil in water for 5 minutes and then steep for another 10 minutes. Apply the liquid to the affected area with cotton swabs.

Afterword: Bringing It All Together

Now that you've finished reading this book, my hope is that it has presented you with many things to think about. First of all, I hope it has eased any fears of your dentist, and given you an understanding of what goes on in a holistic dentist's office such as my own.

So often people think there is something intimidating about going to see a dentist. What I enjoy most is when my patients say, "I like coming here. You talk to me and explain things."

That's the way it should be. I have compassion for and interest in my patients. I think most dentists feel the same way. The problem is that, in dental school, they never teach you how to communicate with your patients.

After reading this book, I want you to be less wary of communicating with your dentist. I want you to be able to say, "Whoa, put down that instrument for a moment, and tell me why you want to cut away my gums."

When he hesitates, I want you to say, "I want to change my diet, I want better ways to deal with this problem. I want my teeth to get better. Let's talk about that first." This will give you what all patients—whether in dental or medical offices—should have: a sense of taking charge of your health.

When I first started researching this book, I got a brand-new text on periodontal disease that was written in 1997. It is 600 pages long, and guess what? There is not one single paragraph in this book about nutrition!

It's all about bone grafting, surgeries, and this and that. Nothing about nutrition. And yet we can successfully cure, or maintain, 90 percent of periodontal cases simply by good nutrition!

I hope that this book helps to wake up the dental industry. We don't need more invasive techniques. What we need is more common sense. Nutritional healing makes more sense to me than rushing into surgery.

We need to become aware that the problems we're seeing in our dental offices are related to problems that doctors are seeing in their medical offices—heart disease, diabetes, and so on. It's common sense to figure out that there is a link, and to treat a dental patient accordingly.

Hopefully, after reading this book, the next time you go to the supermarket you'll think about what you put into your mouth and how it can affect not only your teeth—but your entire body. If your mouth is healthy, your body will be healthy!

If you do eat well and make the dietary, health, and lifestyle changes I've talked about, your mouth will be in great shape—just like the rest of you.

Dr. Victor Zeines is available for consultation regarding any dental questions you may have. He can be reached at 212-813-9461 or 914-657-2322.

Selected References

Chapter 1.
What *Is* Holistic Dentistry?

"Another link between gum disease and heart damage," *Men's Health*, July/August 1998, 34.

Brody, Jane E. "Flossing protects far more than the teeth and gums," *New York Times*, December 19, 1998.

Bronte, Lydia. "Carl Faberge is my dentist," *New Life*, May/June 1999, 19.

"Dental/stroke link," *Bottom Line Health*, October 1998, 6.

Hussar, Christopher. "No more chronic pain," *Alternative Medicine Digest*, 1999, 15:30–34.

Mittelman, Jerry. "What is holistic dentistry?," *New Life*, May/June 1999, 18–19.

"Pearly whites make for happy hearts," *Vegetarian Times*, May 1998, 17.

Stanley, Rhona G. "I followed my dream," *New Life*, May/June 1999, 28–29.

Sternberg, Steve. "Chronic tooth infections can kill more than a smile," *USA Today*, April 14, 1999.

Zeines, Victor. "Your mouth is an indicator of your body's health," *New Life*, May/June 1999, 19–20.

Chapter 2.
Welcome to My Office

Beadall, Alan G. *Clinical Kinesiology*, vols. 1–5, 1980–85.

Gaynor, Mitchell. *Dr. Gaynor's Cancer Prevention Program*, New York: Kensington, 1999.

Lad, Vasant. *Ayurveda: The Science of Self Healing*, Wilmont, WI: Lotus Press, 1990.

Levy, S. and Lehr, C. *Your Body Can Talk*, Prescott, AZ: Hohm Press, 1996.

Maciocia, Giovanni. *Tongue Diagnosis in Chinese Medicine*, Seattle: Eastland Press, 1995.

Moore, Stephen D. "Orange tonsils reveal link to athereosclerosis," *Wall Street Journal*, August 3, 1999.

Muramoto, Naboru. *Healing Ourselves*, Garden City Park, NY: Avery, 1973.

Murray, Michael. *Encyclopedia of Natural Medicine*, Rocklin, CA: Prima, 1991.

Wolf, Harri. *Applied Iridology*, 1:19–31, San Diego, CA: National Iridology Research Association, 1979.

Zeines, Victor. *The Body's Early Warning System*, Holistic Happenings, 1981.

Chapter 4.
Knocking Out Those Pesky Bacteria

Appleton, N. *Healthy Bones*, Garden City Park, NY: Avery, 1991.

Lee, Royal. *Assorted Lectures, 1923–1963*, Palmyra, WI: Lee Foundation for Nutritional Research.

Lust, John. *The Herb Book*, New York: Bantam, 1974.

Moss, Mark E., Auinger, Peggy, and Lamphear, Bruce. *Journal of the American Medical Association*, June 23, 1999.

Page, Melvin and Abrams, L. *Your Body Is Your Best Doctor*, New Canaan, CT: Keats, 1972, 188–203.

Pediatric Dentistry, 21:109–13, April 1999.

Price, Weston. *Nutrition and Physical Degeneration*, Price–Pottinger Nutrition Foundation, 1939.

Scalzo, R. *The Naturopathic Handbook of Herbal Formulas*, Kivaki Press, 1994.

Steggerda, Morris. *Maya Indians of Yucatan*, Publication 531, Carnegie Institute, Washington, DC, 1941.

Sternberg, Steve. "Chronic tooth infections can kill more than a smile," *USA Today*, April 14, 1999.

Tobe, J. *Proven Herbal Remedies*, Pyramid Books, 1973.

Weil, Andrew. "Ask Dr. Weil," *Self Healing*, February 1999, 4.

Zeines, Victor. "Nutrition eases dental problems," *Journal of Nutritional Consultants*, May 1980.

Chapter 5.
The High Price of Convenience

"Gum disease: Do you need surgery?," *Consumer Reports*, February 1996, 60.

Page, Melvin. *Your Body Is Your Best Doctor*, New Canaan, CT: Keats, 1972, 112–15.

Weiss, Ervin I. et al. "Inhibiting interspecies coaggregation of plaque bacteria with a cranberry juice constituent," *Journal of the American Dental Association*, 129:1719–23, 1998.

Wilson, T. and Kornman, K. *Fundamentals of Periodontics*, Quintessence Books, 1996, 250.

Zeines. Victor, "Nutrition eases dental problems," *Journal of Nutritional Consultants*, May 1980.

Chapter 6.
Tooth Decay and Toothaches

Chapman, J. B. *The Biochemical Handbook*, Formur, 1976, 27.

Griffith, H. Winter. *Complete Guide to Medical Tests*, Tuscon, AZ: Fisher Books, 1988.

Harper, H. *Review of Physiological Chemistry*, 16th ed., Lange, 1977, 202.

Page, Melvin. *Your Body Is Your Best Doctor*, New Canaan, CT: Keats, 1972, 196–99.

Chapter 7.
Saving Your Gums

Packer, Lester and Colman, Carol. *The Antioxidant Miracle*, New York: Wiley, 1999.

Pressman, Alan H. *The Complete Idiot's Guide to Vitamins and Minerals*, New York: Alpha/Macmillan, 1997.

Romano, Rita. *Dining in the Raw*, New York: Kensington, 1992.

Chapter 8.
Good Foods, Bad Foods

Baum, Seth J. *The Total Guide to a Healthy Heart*, New York: Kensington, 1999.

Folkers, K. and Wolaniuk, A. "Research on coenzyme Q10 in clinical medicine and immunomodulation," *Drugs Under Experimental and Clinical Research*, 11:539–45, 1985.

Hansen, L.L. et al. "Gingival and leucocytic deficiencies of coenzyme Q10 in patients with periodontal disease," *Research Communications in Chemical Pathological Pharmacology*, 14:729–38, 1976.

Chapter 9.
The Best Vitamins for Dental Health

Pressman, Alan H. *The Complete Idiot's Guide to Vitamins and Minerals*, New York: Alpha/Macmillan, 1997.

Wilkinson, E. G. et al. "Adjunctive treatment of periodontal disease with coenzyme Q10," *Research Communications in Chemical Pathological Pharmacology*, 14:715–19, 1976.

Zucker, Martin. "CoQ10: The newest weapon against gum disease," *Let's Live*, December 1998.

Chapter 10.
Minding Your Minerals

Pressman, Alan H. *The Complete Idiot's Guide to Vitamins and Minerals*, New York: Alpha/Macmillan, 1997.

Romano, Rita. *Dining in the Raw*, New York: Kensington, 1992.

Chapter 11.
Those Sugar Time Blues

Blaylock, Russell. *Excitotoxins: The Taste That Kills*, Sante Fe: Health Press, 1994.

Bottom Line Health, April 1998, 12.

Burros, Marian. "Fears about fat prompt a call to improve the labeling on sugar," *New York Times*, August 4, 1999.

Gittleman, Ann Louise. *How to Stay Young and Healthy in a Toxic World*, Los Angeles: Keats, 1999.

Hunt, Douglas. *No More Cravings*, New York: Warner Books, 1987.

Journal of Nutrition, September 28, 1999, 1442–49.

McCarthy, Laura Flynn. "Much sweeter than sugar, but as safe?" *Rx Remedy*, July/August 1999, 10–11.

Sahelian, Ray and Gates, Donna. *The Stevia Cookbook*, Garden City Park, NY: Avery, 1999.

"Soothe your sweet tooth—naturally," *Whole Foods*, June 1999, 66.

"Vital statistics," *Health*, April 1999, 22.

Chapter 12.
Fluoride: A Blessing or a Curse?

Brown, Ellen Hodgson and Hansen, Richard T. *The Key to Ultimate Health*, Fullerton, CA: Advanced Health Research Publishing, 1998.

Consumer Reports, January 1990.

Galland, Leo. *The Four Pillars of Healing*, New York: Random House, 1997.

Gittleman, Ann Louise. *How to Stay Young and Healthy in a Toxic World*, Los Angeles: Keats, 1999.

Huemer, Richard P. "Fluoride: Fact, fiction, and fear," *Let's Live*, March 1999, 29–31.

Laudan, Larry. *Danger Ahead: The Risks You Really Face on Life's Highway*, New York: Wiley, 1997.

Levy, Thomas. "Fluoridation: Paving the road . . . to the final solution," *Extraordinary Science*, January/March 1994.

Null, Gary. "The fluoridation fiasco," *Townsend Letter for Doctors & Patients*, August/September 1996, 56.

Sims, Shari. "Testing the waters," *Rx Remedy*, July/August 1999, 22.

Steingraber, Sandra. *Living Downstream: An Ecologist Looks at Cancer and the Environment*, Reading, MA: Addison-Wesley, 1997.

Upton, Arthur C. and Graber, Eden. eds. *Staying Healthy in a Risky Environment: The New York University Medical Center Family Guide*, New York: Simon & Schuster, 1993.

Weil, Andrew. *Natural Health, Natural Medicine*, Rev. ed., Boston: Houghton Mifflin, 1995.

Chapter 13.
Remedies From a Natural Dentist

Estafan, D. et al. "Clinical efficacy of a herbal toothpaste," *Journal of Clinical Dentistry*, 9:31–33, 1998.

Burton Goldberg Group, *Alternative Medicine*, Puyallup, WA: Future Medicine Publishing, 1995.

Gultz, J. et al. "An *in vivo* comparison of the antimicrobial activities of three mouth rinses," *Journal of Clinical Dentistry*, 9:43–45, 1998.

Gultz, J. et al. *Antimicrobial Activity Produced by Five Commercially Available Dentifrices, The*, paper presented at New York University College of Dentistry, October 1997.

Gultz, J. et al. *Clinical Efficacy of an Herbal Mouth Rinse*, paper presented at New York University College of Dentistry, March 1998.

Kaim, J. M. et al. "An *in vitro* investigation of the antimicrobial activity of an herbal mouth rinse," *Journal of Clinical Dentistry*, 9:46–48, 1998.

Lust, John. *The Herb Book*, New York: Bantam, 1974.

Mindell, Earl. *Herbs*, New York: Fireside/Simon & Schuster, 1992.

Soule, Deb. *The Roots of Healing: A Woman's Book of Herbs*, New York: Citadel Press, 1995.

Chapter 14.
Bad Breath and Cold Sores

Halpert, Marcella. "In order to save your health you must save your teeth," *New Life*, May/June, 1999.

Kluger, Jeffrey. "Scents and sensibilities," *Discover*, June 1996, 98–101.

Chapter 15.
The Root Canal Controversy

Atkins, Robert. *Secrets of the Atkins Center,* September 1996.

Cavalleri et al. "Comparison of calcium hydroxide and calcium oxide for intercanal medication," *G. Ital. Endodonzia,* 4(3):8–13, 1990.

Georgopolou, M. et al. "In vitro evaluation of the effectiveness of calcium hydroxide and paramonochlorophenol on anaerobic bacteria from the root canal," *Endo. Dent. Traumatol,* 9(6):249–53, December 1993.

Ingle, J. I. and Bakland, L. K. *Endodontics,* 4th ed., Malvern, PA: Williams & Wilkins, 1994.

Meinig, George. *Root Canal Cover Up,* Ojai, CA: Bion Publishing, 1994.

Messing, J. J. and Stock, C. J. R. *Color Atlas of Endodontics,* St. Louis: Wolfe Medical Publications, 1988, 178–80.

Chapter 16.
Cavitation: The Hole in Your Jaw

Bouquot, J. E. and McMahon, R. E. "Ischemic osteonecrosis in facial pain syndromes: A review of NICO (neuralgia-inducing cavitational osteonecrosis) based on experience with more than 2,000 patients," *TM Diary,* 8:32–39, 1996.

Breiner, Mark A. *Whole-Body Dentistry,* Fairfield, CT: Quantum Health Press, 1999.

Glueck, C. J. et al. "Thrombofilia, hyperfibrinolysis, alveolar osteonecrosis of the jaws," *Oral Surgery, Oral Medicine, Oral Pathology,* 81:557–66, 1996.

Inabinet, Carolyn. "A bone of contention—cavitations vs. osteonecrosis," *Arizona Networking News,* December 1998/January 1999.

Laura Lee interview with George Meinig, DDS, and Dr. M. LaMarche: "Cavitations and root canals," *Townsend Letter for Doctors & Patients,* August/September 1996.

Stockton, Susan. *Beyond Amalgam,* North Port, FL: Nature's Publishing, 1998.

Chapter 17.
Are Your Fillings Killing You?

Brun, R. "Epidemiology of contact dermatitis in Geneva," *Contact Dermatitis*, 1:214–17, 1975.

Djerassi, E. and Berova, N. "The possibilities of allergic reactions from silver amalgam restorations," *Intern. Dent. J.*, 19(4):481–88, 1969.

Eggleston, D. "Effects of dental amalgam and nickel alloys on T-lymphocytes," *Journal of Prosthetic Dentistry*, 51:617–23, August 1984.

Eggleston, D. et al. "Correlation of amalgam with mercury in brain tissue," *Journal of Prosthetic Dentistry*, 58:704–7, 1987.

Gary Null Newsletter, Summer 1978.

Hahn, L. J. et al. "Whole body imaging of the distribution of mercury released from dental silver fillings into monkey tissues," *FASEB Journal*, 4:3256–60, November 1990.

Huggins, Hal A. *It's All in Your Head: The Link Between Mercury and Illness*, Garden City Park, NY: Avery, 1993.

Huggins, Hal A. *Serum Compatibility Testing: A Crucial Methodology for Modern Dentistry*, Colorado Springs: Huggins Diagnostics, 1989.

Nylander, M. et al. "Mercury concentrations in the human brain and kidneys in relation to exposure from dental fillings," *Swedish Dental Journal*, 11:179–87, 1987.

Royal, F. Fuller. "Are dentists contributing to our declining health?," *Townsend Letter for Doctors & Patients*, May 1990, 311–14.

Rudner et al. "Epidemiology of contact dermatitis in North America," *Archives of Dermatology*, 108:537–40, 1973.

Vimy, M. et al. "Glomerular filtration impairment by mercury released from silver fillings in sheep," *Physiologist*, 33(4):A–94, August 1990.

Wenstrup, D. et al. "Trace element imbalances in isolated subcellular fractions of Alzheimer's disease brain," *Brain Research*, 553:125–31, 1990.

Ziff, Sam, Ziff, Michael F. and Hanson, Mats. *Dental Mercury Detox*, 6th ed., Orlando, FL: BioProbe, 1997.

Chapter 18.
Secrets of a Perfect Smile

Breiner, Mark A. *Whole-Body Dentistry,* Fairfield, CT: Quantum Health Press, 1999.

Brown, Ellen Hodgson, and Hansen, Richard T. *The Key to Ultimate Health,* Fullerton, CA: Advanced Health Research Publishing, 1998.

Kennedy, David. *How to Save Your Teeth,* Delaware, OH: Health Action Press, 1993.

Stay, Flora Parsa. *The Complete Book of Dental Remedies,* Garden City Park, NY: Avery, 1996.

Chapter 19.
From Magnets to Muscle Testing

Breiner, Mark A. *Whole-Body Dentistry,* Fairfield, CT: Quantum Health Press, 1999.

Davis, Albert Roy, and Rawls, Jr., Walter C. *The Magnetic Effect,* Kansas City, MO: Acres U.S.A., 7th printing, 1993.

Levy, Susan L. and Lehr, Carol. *Your Body Can Talk,* Prescott, AZ: Hohm Press, 1996.

Wolfe, Bill. "Preventive dentistry and you: Treating TMJ syndrome," *Let's Live,* March 1990, 75.

Chapter 20.
Homeopathic Healers

Stay, Flora Parsa. *The Complete Book of Dental Remedies,* Garden City Park, NY: Avery, 1996.

Wolfe, Bill. "Homeopathic treatment of gingivitis," *Biological Therapy,* 14(3):259, 1996.

Yasgur, Jay. *Yasgur's Homeopathic Dictionary and Holistic Health Reference,* Greenville, PA: Van Hoy Publishers, 1998.

Chapter 21.
The Pick of the Crop

Crawford, Amanda McQuade. *Herbal Remedies for Women,* Rocklin, CA: Prima, 1997.

Lust, John. *The Herb Book,* New York: Bantam, 1974.

Murray, Michael T. *The Healing Power of Herbs,* Rocklin, CA: Prima, 2d ed., 1995.

Pitman, Vicki. *Herbal Medicine,* Rockport, MA: Element, 1994.

Soule, Deb. *The Roots of Healing,* New York: Carol, 1995.

Tierra, Michael. *The Way of Chinese Herbs,* New York: Pocket Books, 1998.

Tierra, Michael. *The Way of Herbs,* New York: Pocket Books, 1998.

Resource Section

Companies

The following companies have a number of products listed in this resource section. Companies with only one product listed have their toll-free numbers and websites listed along with their products.

Body Wise
1-800-830-9596
www.bodywise.com

Carlson® Laboratories
800-323-4141
www.carlsonlabs.com

Gaia Herbs, Inc.
1-800-831-7780
www.gaiaherbs.com

Jarrow Formulas™
1-800-726-0886
www.jarrow.com

MegaFood
800-848-2542
www.megafood.com

N.E.E.D.S.
1-800-634-1380
www.needs.com

Prevail Corporation
1-800-248-0855
www.prevail.com

Source Naturals®
800-815-2333
www.sourcenaturals.com

Tree of Life®
www.treeoflife.com

Tyler, Inc.
1-800-869-9705
www.tyler-inc.com

Wakunaga of America, Inc.
1-800-421-2998
www.kyolic.com

Supplements

Listed here are nutritional supplements recommended by Dr. Victor Zeines. We have endeavored to find the best companies that carry these supplements. If you cannot find a particular product at your local health food store, please contact the company directly for the names of stores that carry it.

Acidophilus (Probiotics)

Available from the following companies:

Garden of Life
1-800-622-8986

❋ Primal Defense™ HSO™ (Homeostatic Soil Organisms)
Soil-based probiotic containing acidophilus bulgaricus and many other probiotic ingredients. Also contains organic green grass juices and pre-digested PhytoSterol/Sterolins. Available in 500 mg capsules.

Jarrow Formulas™
Jarro-Dophilus™
High potency, non-dairy, multi-strain probiotic. Each 280 mg capsule contains six species of the hardiest of the lactobacilli and bifidobacteria at a potency of 10-15 billion per gram. Jarro-Dophilus™ + FOS (available in capsules and powder).

Prevail®
Inner Ecology™
Intestinal balancing acidophilus formula. Dairy-free. Contains specially prepared *lactobacillus* and *bifidobacteria*. Available in powder form.

Source Naturals®
DDS-1 Acidophilus
Each gram of DDS-1 Acidophilus powder contains at least 10 billion viable cells of freeze-dried DDS-1 acidophilus "friendly" flora at the time of manufacture. Available in capsules and powder.

Life Flora™
Acidophilus/Bifidus Complex. Each 300 mg capsule contains 3 billion viable cells of freeze-dried bifidus and DDS-1 acidophilus. Each 500 mg capsule contains 5 billion viable cells of freeze-dried bifidus and DDS-1 acidophilus. Also available in powder form.

NutraFlora® FOS
NutraFlora is a complex of fructooligosaccharides (FOS)—a group of naturally occurring carbohydrates that are indigestible by humans but serve as "food" for friendly flora, helping to increase their numbers in the body. Available in 1,000 mg tablets and powder form.

Tyler

Enterogenic™ Concentrate
Acidophilus Complex with FOS (fructooligosaccharides). Available in capsule and powder.

Adaptogens

To help shield the body against stress. The ones listed below act synergistically in liver cleansing and are great antioxidants.

Swedish Herbal Institute
1-800-774-9444
www.adaptogen.com

Arctic Root®
Available in tablet form.

Chisandra Adaptogen®
Available in tablet form.

Allergy Relief

For allergy sufferers who can have reduced immune function.
Carlson®
Aler-Key®
Hypoallergenic nutritional support for the allergen sensitive. Two capsules contain 800 mg vitamin C, 300 mg quercetin, 200 mg pantothenic acid, 10 mg vitamin B-2, 10 mg vitamin B-6, and 116 mg calcium.

Alpha Lipoic Acid

Available from the following companies:

Tishcon Corporation
1-800-848-8442

Biosolv™, Lipo-Gel™: Each Softsule® contains 100 mg.of alpha lipoic acid and 100 IU of vitamin E.

Source Naturals®
Alpha Lipoic Acid
For immune system support. Stimulates gluthathione production.
Available in 50 mg, 100 mg and 200 mg tablets.

Amino Acids

Carlson®
Amino Blend
Scientifically balanced formulation of 22 essential and non-essential
amino acids, which are the building blocks of protein. Available in capsules and powder form.

Antioxidants

Available from the following companies:

Body Wise
Super Cell™
Each capsule contains a wide range of antioxidants, including vitamin
C, vitamin E, selenium, green tea leaf extract, L-glutathione, and
more.

MegaFood
ANTIOXIDANT DAILYFOODS® Vitamin, Mineral & Herbal
Formula
Contains vitamins A, C and E, zinc and selenium. DAILYFOODS®
FoodState® nutrients are 100% Whole FOOD and can be taken at
any time throughout the day, even on an empty stomach. Available in
tablet form.

Astragalus Extract

Planetary Formulas®
1-800-606-6226
www.planetaryformulas.com
Full Spectrum™ Astragalus Extract
Each two tablet serving combines 500 mg of standardized astralagus
root extract with 500 mg of whole high grade astragalus root.

Bone and Connective Tissue Enhancement
Available from the following companies:
MegaFood
BONE DAILYFOODS®
Vitamin and mineral formula that provides all the essential skeletal nutrients as found in complex foods. Contains vitamins C, D3, K1, calcium, magnesium, manganese, silicon, and boron. DAILYFOODS® FoodState® nutrients are 100% Whole FOOD and can be taken at any time throughout the day, even on an empty stomach. Available in tablet form.

Source Naturals®
OPC-85™
A potent natural antioxidant derived from the bark of the European costal pine *(Pinus maritima)* that helps to maintain the integrity of collagen and elastin, two important constituents of connective tissue. Available in 50 and 100 mg tablets.

Bone Balance™
Contains a 1-1 ratio of calcium and magnesium along with other bone minerals and soy isoflavones, to provide bone and teeth support. Available in tablet form.

Bromelain

Available from the following companies:

Source Naturals®
Bromelain
Each tablet contains 500 mg of bromelain (2,000 GDU per g).

Calcium

Body Wise
Essential Calcium+®
Calcium in tablet form, which also includes vitamin D_3, vitamin B_6, magnesium, zinc, copper, and other ingredients.

Calcium D-Glucarate

Available from the following companies:

Source Naturals®
Calcium D-Glucarate
Cellular detoxifier. Each tablet contains 500 mg of calcium D-glucarate.

Tyler, Inc.
Calcium D-Glucarate™
Available in 500 mg capsules.

Coenzyme Q10

Available from the following companies:

Body Wise
CoEnzyme Q10+
Each capsule contains 30 mg of CoQ10, 30 mg quercetin, and 30 IU vitamin E.

Carlson Laboratories
Co-Q10
Available in 10 mg, 30 mg, 50 mg and 100 mg soft gels.

Source Naturals®
Coenzyme Q10
Available in 30 mg and100 mg softgels.

Tishcon Corporation (raw goods supplier)
1-800-848-8442
www.tish.com/*www.Q-Gel.com*
This is Dr. Zeines' favorite CoQ10. Hydrosoluble and high bioavailability. Comes in softsules® (soft gels).

Q-Gel®: 15 mg
Q-Gel® Forte: 30 mg
Q-Gel® Plus: with 50 mg alpha lipoic acid and 100 IU natural vitamin E
Q-Gel® Ultra: 60 mg
Carni-Q-Gel®: with 30 mg CoQ10 and 250 mg L-carnitine

Tishcon's CoQ10 products are available from the following companies:

Bio Energy Nutrients (a division of Whole Foods): 1-800-627-7775
Physiologics (a division of Whole Foods): 1-800-765-6775
CountryLife: 1-800-645-5768
Solanova: 1-800-200-0456 (ext 108)
Phytotherapy: 201-891-1104
Nutrimedika: 1-800-688-7462
Swanson: 1-800-437-4148
Jordets: 1-888-816-7676
Epic: 1-800-848-8442
Optimum Health: 1-800-228-1507
Doctor's Preferred: 1-800-304-1708

Fish Oils

Available from the following companies:

Carlson Laboratories
Norwegian Cod Liver Oil
Bottled in liquid form. High in omega-3 and other essential fatty acids and vitamin E. Available in natural and lemon-flavored. Can be mixed into foods.

Norwegian Salmon Oil
Each soft gel contains 1000 mg of salmon oil. Two softgels provide 710 mg of total omega-3 fatty acids, including EPA (Eicosapentaenoic Acid), DHA (Docosahexaenoic Acid), DPA (Docosapentaenoic Acid) and ALA (Alpha-Liolenic Acid).

Super-DHA™
Each soft gel contains 1000 mg of a special blend of fish body oils, including menhaden and sardines, which are high in DHA (Docosahexaenoic Acid) and EPA (Eicosapentaenoic Acid).

Super Omega-3 Fish Oils
Contains a special concentrate of fish body oils from deep, cold-water fish, including mackerel and sardines, which are especially rich in EPA and DHA. Each soft gel provides 570 mg of total omega-3 fatty acids consisting of EPA (Eicosapentaenoic Acid), DHA (Docosahexaenoic Acid), and ALA ((Alpha-Liolenic Acid).

Prevail Corporation
Eskimo-3®
Natural stable fish oil with vitamin E. Each serving of three soft gels contains 500 mg of omega-3, 240 mg of EPA, 160 mg of DHA, and 6.7 IU of vitamin E.

Flaxseed Oil

Available from the following companies:

Tree of Life®
High Lignan Flax Oil
Contains all the antioxidants of their original Organic Flax Oil plus the added benefits of high fiber lignans. Bottled in liquid form. Available in health food stores.

Garlic

Wakunaga of America
Kyolic® Aged Garlic Extract (AGE)
The most scientifically researched garlic product in the world (over 220 studies). Available in capsules as well as in liquid form (that can be added to food).

Glutathione

Available from the following companies:

Carlson® Laboratories
Glutathione Booster™
Provides the body with the nutrients needed to elevate or maintain healthy glutathione and glutathione peroxidase levels. Each capsule contains vitamins C and E, riboflavin (vitamin B-2), selenium, n-acetyl cysteine, milk thistle extract (silymarin), garlic, alpha lipoic, L-glutamine, L-glycine, asparagus concentrate, and glutathione.

Prevail Corporation
GSH Cell Support
Contains reduced L-glutathione and anthocyanidins in capsule form.

Source Naturals®
L-Glutathione
Available in 50 mg tablets

Chem-Defense™
Molybdenum/glutathione complex. Helps to remove toxins from the body. Each orange-flavored tablet contains 1.6 mg of riboflavin (as 2.25 mg flavin mononucleotide [Coenzymated™]), 120 mcg of molybdenum (as molybdenum aspartate citrate) and 50 mg of glutathione. Taken sublingually (under the tongue) for direct absorption into the bloodstream.

Tyler, Inc.
Recancostat® 400
Each capsule contains 400 mg of reduced L-glutathione along with beet root, black currant, bilberry, elderberry, L-cysteine, and other ingredients. Terrific precursor for glutathione in the body.

Green Tea Extract

Source Naturals®
Green Tea Extract
Each tablet contains 100 mg of standardized, patented Polyphenon 60™ green tea extract, providing at least 65 mg of polyphenols.

Immune System Support

Body Wise
AG-Immune™
Dietary supplement for a healthy immune system. Two capsules contain 300 mg Immune Enhancer™ AG (arabinogalactan), 100 mg Ai/E^{10}™ (Whey), 50 mg astragalus root, 50 mg maitake mushroom extract 4.1, and other ingredients. This is the only Ai/E^{10}™ formulation that combines these immune-boosting ingredients.

Moducare Sterinol™
A wonderful new immune enhancer that is now widely available. Moducare Sterinol is a patented blend of plant sterols and sterolins that possess a powerful immune system enhancement. It has been shown to increase Natural Killer Cell activity in your body and mouth for anti-inflammation and infection. Thousands of research studies have been published worldwide on plant sterols and sterolins, including 140 double-blind trials in humans. Available from the following companies:

Moducare Sterinol
877-297-7332
www.moducare.com

Natural Balance
800-833-8737
www.naturalbalance.com

(In Canada) Purity Life Health Products
800-265-2615

L-Glutamine

N.E.E.D.S.
Available in capsules, tablets and powder.

Liver Support

Available from the following companies:

Prevail®
Metabolic Liver Formula™
Contains 80% silymarin with Plant Enzymes™, black radish root, dandelion root, beet leaf, kelp and other effective ingredients. Available in capsules.

Source Naturals®
Liver Guard™
Contains lipoic acid, silymarin and N-acetyl cysteine (NAC) to support healthy liver function. Also contains herbs for cleansing the liver as well as choline and inositol for preventing fat from depositing in the liver. Available in tablets.

Mail Order

N.E.E.D.S
1-800-634-1380
www.needs.com
N.E.E.D.S. carries a full line of quality supplements from top companies.

MSM

Carlson®
MSM Sulfur
Each capsule contains 1,000 mg of MSM (methylsulfonylmethane), providing 334 mg of organic dietary sulfur.

Multivitamin and Mineral Formulations

Available from the following companies:

Body Wise
Right Choice®
Comprehensive multiple in two formulations: AM for the morning and PM for the night. Scientifically designed for maximum effect. Available in tablet form.

MegaFood
LIFESTYLE™ DAILYFOODS® Vitamin, Mineral & Herbal Formula
This unique formulation delivers nutrients in the FoodState® for maximum utilization. Recent scientific studies have proven that nutrients function at their peak when consumed as they naturally occur in food. Because MegaFood's formulas are food, they are particularly effective. DAILYFOODS® FoodState® nutrients are 100% Whole FOOD and can be taken at any time throughout the day, even on an empty stomach. Available in tablet form.

Pycnogenol

Source Naturals®
Pycnogenol®
Proanthocyanidin Complex. Available in 25 mg, 50 mg, 75 mg, and 100 mg tablets.

Pyconogenol® Complex
Antioxidant Formula. Combines pycnogenol and proanthodyn (grape seed extract), antioxidants and plantioxidants (plant-derived antioxidants). Available in tablet form.

Selenium

Available from the following companies:

Carlson®

Selenium
Yeast-free. Each capsule contains organically bound selenium from L-selenomethionine, providing 200 mcg of selenium.

E-Sel
Natural-source vitamin E and organic selenium. Two soft gels contain 400 IU of vitamin E (d-alpha tocopheryl acetate derived from soybean oil) and 100 mcg of selenium (from L-selenomethione).

Source Naturals®
Selenomax®
Contains selenium from Selenomax® high selenium yeast. Available in 100 mcg and 200 mcg tablets.

Vitamins A & D

Carlson®
Vitamins A and D_3
Each soft gel contains 10,000 IU of natural source vitamin A and 400 IU of natural source vitamin D_3 from fish liver oil.

Vitamin B Complex

Available from the following companies:

Carlson®
B-Compleet™
Provides all the B-vitamins plus vitamin C in a balanced formulation. Available in tablets.

Source Naturals®
Coenzymate™ B Complex
Contains coenzymes along with a full range of B-vitamins and CoQ10.

Available in orange or peppermint flavored tablets that are taken sublingually (under the tongue) for direct absorption into the bloodstream.

Vitamin C

Available from the following companies:

Body Wise
Beta C™
Comprehensive vitamin C in tablet form.

Carlson®
Mild-C Chewable
Buffered form of chewable vitamin C that is non-acidic and gentle to the teeth. Each orange and tangerine flavored tablet supplies 250 mg of vitamin C and 28 mg of calcium.

MegaFood
Complex C
Vitamin C as found in food, is a very complex nutrient of which ascorbic acid is only one factor. Complex C DAILYFOOD® contains all the food factors, such as bioflavonoids, that occur in food and enhance its effectiveness. DAILYFOODS® FoodState® nutrients are 100% Whole FOOD and can be taken at any time throughout the day, even on an empty stomach. Available in 250 mg tablets.

Source Naturals®
C-500
Each tablet provides 500 mg of vitamin C (ascorbic acid) and 50 mg of rose hips.

C-1000 Time Release
Provides a gradual release over a prolonged period of time. Each tablet provides 1,000 mg of vitamin C (ascorbic acid) and 100 mg of rose hips.

Wellness C-1000™
Each tablet contains 1,000 mg of vitamin C and several sources of bioflavonoids and alpha-lipoic acid.

Vitamin D

Available from the following companies:

Moss Nutrition
1-800-851-5444
Bio-D-Mulsion
An oil in water emulsion in which vitamin D has been dispersed. Each drop supplies 400 IU of emulsified vitamin D. If you wish to have your dentist or physician inquire about this product, they can call Moss Nutrition.

Carlson®
Vitamin D_3
Natural source vitamin D_3 from fish liver oil. Available in 400 IU and 1,000 IU soft gels.

Vitamin E

Available from the following companies:

Carlson®
d-Alpha Gems™
Each tiny soft gel contains 400 IU of vitamin E (d-alpha tocopherol acetate).

E-Gems® Plus
Each soft gel contains vitamin E derived from soybean oil, supplying alpha-tocopherol plus mixed tocopherols. Available in three strengths: 200 IU, 400 IU and 800 IU.

Jarrow Formulas
Oil E
Vitamin E as 100% natural form d-alpha tocopherol with mixed tocopherols. Available in 400 IU and 600 IU soft gels.

MegaFood
E & Selenium DAILYFOODS®

In foods, vitamin E and selenium are always found together. Vitamin E doesn't work without the presence of selenium and vice versa. This combination offers these two important nutrients as they naturally occur in food, and therefore provides maximum protection. DAILY-FOODS® FoodState® nutrients are 100% Whole FOOD and can be taken at any time throughout the day, even on an empty stomach. Each tablet contains 100 IU of vitamin E and 100 mg of selenium.

Source Naturals®
Vitamin E

Each softgel contains 400 IU of natural vitamin E (d-alpha tocopherol) and 67 mg of mixed tocopherols (d-beta, d-gamma, and d-delta). In a base of soybean oil.

Tocotrienol Antioxidant Complex™

Each softgel contains a total of 34 mg of tocotrienols (29.8 mg gamma-tocotrienol, 3 mg alpha-tocotrienol, and 1.3 mg delta-tocotrienol) and 100 IU of vitamin E (d-alpha tocopherol).

Zinc

Available from the following companies:

Carlson® Laboratories
Zine

Contains zinc from zinc gluconate in 15 mg and 50 mg tablets.

Jarrow Formulas™
Zinc Balance 15™

A synergistic combination of OptiZinc™ brand zinc monomethionate and copper gluconate in a 15:1 zinc/copper ratio. Each capsule contains 15 mg of zinc (as monomethionine) and 1 mg of copper (as gluconate).

Source Naturals®
OptiZinc®
Each tablet contains 30 mg of zinc (from 150 mg of OptiZinc® zinc monomethionine)

Detoxification

Gaia Herbs, Inc.
Supreme Cleanse™ Internal Cleansing Program
Contains certified organic and ecologically wild-crafted herbs that are specifically selected and formulated to work synergistically within the body to clear accumulated toxins and wastes.

High Tech Health
1-800-794-5355
www.hightechhealth.com
Thermal Life® Far Infrared Therapy Sauna
A marvelous detoxification sauna (described in this book) that doesn't need any water and can be moved anywhere in the home or apartment. Unit sizes available for 1-5 persons.

Tyler
Mercury Detox™
Contains specific nutrients and cofactors utilized by detoxification pathways for mercury and other heavy metals as well as amino acids that protect the central nervous system from mercury toxicity. Two capsules provide the following: 400 mg N-Acetyl-Cysteine, 200 mg L-Methionine, 200 mg L-Leucine, 200 mg L-Valine, 200 mg L-Isoleucine, 150 mg Taurine, 100 mg L-Glutathione, 25 mg Magnesium, 75 IU Vitamin E, and 150 mcg Selenium.

Herbs

Because the list of herbs that Dr. Zeines recommends is too lengthy to fit into this resource section, Dr. Zeines has selected the following top five herb companies whose products you can rely on for safety and potency.

Gaia Herbs
1-800-831-7780
www.gaiaherbs.com
Founded by Ric Scalzo. They cultivate their own certified organic crop on 200 acres.

Herbalists and Alchemists
1-800-611-8235
www.Herbalist-Alchemist.com
Founded by herbalist David Winston. Provides some of the highest quality herbal tinctures and herbal products available in the United States.

Herbal Pharm
1-800-348-4372
www.Herb-Pharm.com
Founded by Ed Smith, "Herbal Ed." They organically cultivate and ecologically wildcraft their own herbs and make a superb line of herbal extracts.

Planetary Herbs/Formulas
1-800-777-5677
www.planetherbs.com
Dr. Michael Tierra, OMD, L.Ac., is one of the foremost authorities on herbal medicine in North America and has had a clinical practice for 30 years. He is the product formulator for Planetary Formulas and is an internationally recognized authority on the world's herbal traditions.

Homeopathic

Boericke & Tafel, Inc. (B&T)
1-800-876-9505
bandt@boericke.com (e-mail)
A recommended homeopathic company, founded in 1835, B&T has been a pioneer in the field of homeopathy. They have been conducting double blind, placebo controlled clinical studies for years. Their medicines are made in accordance with the FDA's Good Manufacturing Practices.

Whole Food Suppliers

Bottled Water

Mountain Valley Water
1-800-643-1501
A fine, slightly alkaline water, bottled in glass from a pure, natural spring. Available in 5 gallon glass bottles and smaller sizes for easy-carrying.

Culinary Herbs and Spices

Frontier Herbs
1-800-669-3275
Provides high quality herbs and spices as well as various herbal products.

Flaxseeds

Health From The Sun
1-800-447-2229
FiPro FLAX™
Organic ground flaxseeds combined with fermented soy meal and other ingredients. Crunchy texture and delicious, nutty taste. Sprinkle on salads, cereal, soup and pasta. Available in healthfood stores.

Grains

Lundberg Family Farms
530-882-4550 (ext. 319)
www.lundberg.com
Grower and marketer of organic rice and rice products. This is Dr. Zeines' favorite rice company. They have an amazing variety of rices, rice cakes, etc. Reliable quality.

Powdered Green Drink

Wakunaga
Kyo-Green®
A combination of organically grown barley and wheat grasses, kelp, chlorella and brown rice. Two teaspoons provide the nutrients of a serving of deep green leafy vegetables.

Poultry

Sheltons Poultry, Inc.
1-800-541-1844
Free-range and no added antibiotics. Available in natural food stores.

Seafood

Available from the following companies:

Capilano Pacific
1-877-391-WILD (9453)
www.capilanopacific.com
Wildfish™
This company is a wonderful source for wild-caught salmon. Most of the salmon available in restaurants and stores are farm-raised. Usually this means medications such as antibiotics have been added to the feed, as well as synthetic coloring. Wild-caught salmon has none of these problems and a higher level of omega-3 fatty acids and much less fat than farm-raised salmon. It tastes better as well. Also available: halibut, tuna and lox without any added chemicals.

New World Marketing Group
203-221-8008
Sardines
Packed in pure virgin olive oil and virgin olive oil with garlic. Very high in omega-3 fatty acids. They also have water-packed sardines which contain less sodium. Available in natural foods stores.

Stevia

Wisdom of the Ancients®
1-800-899-9908
www.wisdomherbs.com
Natural sweetener made from whole leaf Stevia *(Stevia rebaudiana Berton)* 6:1 concentrated extract. This is a dentist's wish come true—a natural sweetener that is good for the body and does no harm to the teeth. Available in concentrated tablets, liquid, and as a tea.

Teas (Green)

Available from the following companies:

Great Eastern Sun
1-800-334-5809
www.great-eastern-sun.com

Haiku® Organic Japanese Teas
Organic Original Sencha Green Tea: the finest grade of green leaf tea available, made from the tender young leaves of selected tea bushes, cut at the peak of their flavor, rolled, steamed, and briefly dried. Contains 100% Nagata Japanese Organic Sencha Green Tea Leaves and Buds. Available in tea bags and bulk.

Organic Original Hojicha Roated Green Tea: lower in caffeine than Sencha, Hojicha has a subtle smoky and rich flavor that is quite different from that of Sencha. Contains 100% Nagata Japanese Organic Hojicha Roasted Green Tea Leaves and Stems. Available in tea bags and bulk.

Maitake Products, Inc.
1-800-747-7418
www.maitake.com
Mai Green™ Tea
Contains organically grown maitake mushroom and premier Japanese green tea (matcha) leaves. Low in caffeine. Available in tea bags.

Triple Leaf Tea, Inc.
1-800-552-7448
Authentic traditional Chinese medicinal teas in tea bags, including different varieties of green tea. Triple Leaf has a wonderful natural method of decaffeinating green tea without using any chemical solvents. If you drink a lot of green tea and don't want caffeine, this is an ideal tea to use.

T Salon & Emporium
1-888-NYCTEAS (692-8327)
tsalon@interport.net (e-mail)
T Salon distributes, mail orders, and retails gourmet blended teas, organic greens, and specialty black teas. Favorites are Japanese Berry, Whispering Heaven, Tibetan Tiger, Mandarin Earl Grey, and Vanilla Chai. Their teas can be found at Whole Foods Supermarkets located nationwide, and at popular four-star restaurants.

Tree of Life®
www.treeoflife.com
There are many fine health food stores all over the country that carry top-notch products. Many stores are supplied by an excellent company known as Tree of Life, a distributor of high quality natural foods and supplements at moderate prices. Tree of Life's supplements are pharmaceutical grade, exceeding the current Good Manufacturing Standards as well as passing all tests performed by the USP (United States Pharmacopia). When shopping at health food stores, you can ask for Tree of Life products. If a store doesn't carry a particular product, they can order it for you.

Tree of Life Frozen Organic Vegetables
These are ideal to stock in your freezer if you don't always have access or organic vegetables:
Broccoli Cuts
Green Peas
Spinach

Tree of Life Frozen Fruit
Organic fruits are loaded with nutrients. These are often difficult to obtain:
Strawberries
Blueberries
Raspberries

Tree of Life Frozen Smoothie Makers
Fresh-frozen chunks of 100% organic fruit. Ideal for juicing.
Banana, Rasberry, Strawberry

Tree of Life Organic Tamari and Shoyu
Made from organic soybeans and wheat. Excellent for steamed vegetables and fish.
Shoyu
Wheat-Free Tamari

Tree of Life Organic Extra Virgin Olive Oil
Bella Via Organic Extra Virgin Olive Oil
Made from the first pressing of 100% organic olives imported from the Andalusia region of Spain.

Tree of Life Organic Almond Butter
Avalable in two ways—creamy and crunchy—in glass jars.
Organic almonds are a good source of B-vitamins, vitamin E, essential fatty acids, calcium, and an array of other important minerals, as well as a substantial amount of protein.

Tree of Life Pasta Sauce
Original and Salt-Free—in glass jars.
This organic pasta sauce is made from vine-ripened, specially selected premium tomatoes that are grown for their sweetness and flavor.

Wine

If you like to have an occasional glass of wine, this is a safe and enjoyable way to do it.

Frey Vineyards
1-800-760-3739
Organic wines with no sulfites or pesticides.

La Rocca Vineyards
1-800-808-9463
www.laroccavineyards.com
Certified organic white and red wines that are sulfite-free.

Dental Resources

Dental Products

Available from the following companies:

Woodstock Natural Products, Inc.
The Natural Dentist™
1-800-615-6895
Toothpastes and mouth rinses, formulated by Dr. Zeines, containing soothing herbs and no alcohol, sugar, or harsh chemicals. These products have been clinically proven to kill germs that cause gum disease.
Toothpaste: mint, cinnamon and fluoride-free mint
Mouth rinse: mint, cinnamon, cherry-flavored

Peelu U.S.A.
1-800-457-3358
The fibers and extracts of the Peelu tree have been used for centuries in Asia and in the Middle East for dental care. Peelu products are sugar-free, with no artificial sweeteners or perservatives, no chemicals or abrasives, and no animal testing.
Peelu Dental Fibers: finely ground, easy-to-apply powder that cleans and brightens teeth. Available in peppermint, spearmint, or mint-free flavors.

Desert Essence®
1-888-476-8647
www.desertessence.com
Oral Care Collection
A complete line of antiseptic and cleansing oral care products using tea tree oil for deep cleaning and disinfecting of teeth and gums. All products are animal and eco-friendly and made without artificial colors, sweeteners or harsh abrasives.

Natural Tea Tree Oil Toothpaste: combats plaque with baking soda and tea tree oil; available in four flavors: fennel, ginger, mint and wintergreen with neem (Ayurvedic extract known to promote oral health).
Tea Tree Oil Dental Floss: creates a germ-free mouth and cleans between teeth
Tea Tree Oil Dental Tape: provides same benefit as floss with a wider ribbon
Tea Tree Oil Dental Pics: cleans between teeth with antiseptic power
Tea Tree Oil Mouthwash: spearmint flavored
Tea Tree Oil Breath Freshener: contains natural and organic essential oils

Removal of Mercury Amalgam Fillings

To find a dentist who can safely remove mercury fillings, contact:

International Academy of Oral Medicine and Toxicology
Michael F. Ziff, D.D.S. Executive Director
P.O. Box 608531
Orlando, FL 32860
407-298-2450
(mercury-free dentists and physicians)

Special Resource Section

Household Cleansers

Available from the following companies:

N.E.E.D.S.
Allens Naturally: A full line of toxin-free household cleansers, including dishwashing and laundry detergents and all-purpose cleaners.

E Cover®
1-800-440-4925
Leading manufacturer of environmentally safe and toxic free household cleaning products. Their line includes dish and laundry products and a full range of household cleansers. Available in health food stores

Juicer

Miracle Exclusives, Inc.
1-800-645-6360
www.miracleexclusives.com
Stainless Steel Juice Extractor (Model MJ 7000-1)
This is a relatively small machine (only 14" high) that is very effective and easy to clean. Hammacher Schlemmer Institute has rated this juice extractor the best for its quality of juice, ease of use, ease of cleaning and construction. Miracle Exclusives has a full line of juicers and a soy milk-making machine.

Grinding Mill

Miracle Mill (Model ME821)
Stainless steel grinder for a wide variety of seeds and grains—including flax and soy beans. Convenient dial provides a range of adjustments from coarse to very fine grind.

Mail Order

N.E.E.D.S.
1-800-634-1380
www.needs.com
An excellent source for top-notch products, including the following:
Aireox Air Purifier (Model 45): removes mold spores, pollen dust, formaldehyde, and more.
Aireox Car Air Purifier (Model 22): an unusual purifier for the car.

Easy Mixer: battery operated mixer that effectively combines powders with liquids.

Elite Shower Filter and Massager: for removing chlorine, heavy metals and bacteria.

Teslar Watch: "The watch that protects" you from many unrecognized dangers of electromagnetic fields produced by cell phones, computers, televisions, telephones, automobiles, fluorescent lights, etc. By adding the Teslar chip to the watch, your Teslar not only tells time but also protects you from harmful ELF's. According to Dr. Doris Rapp, M.D., Dr. John Upledger, D.O., Dr. Valerie Hunt, Ph.D., and Dr. Scott Morley, M.D. (M.A.) "the Teslar watch performs as advertised".

Relaxation and Healing Aid

Sounds True
1-800-333-9185
www.soundstrue.com
Breathing: The Master Key to Self Healing
Recording by Andrew Weil, M.D. (available on CDs or cassettes)
Breathing is an ancient and useful way to relax and actually influence the immune system in a positive way.

Water Filter

High Tech Health, Inc.
1-800-794-5355
http://*www.hightechhealth.com*
Ionizer Plus
A very effective water filter. It provides superior water filtration to 1/10 of a micron (below bacteria levels) and ultraviolet to eliminate viruses. The greatest benefit of this filtration system is its ability to ionize minerals in water, thereby increasing the mineral bioavailability and the PH. This is an execllent method of eliminating digestive and other problems caused by over-acidity. The machine is ideal because it allows you to adjust the alkaline level of the water you drink, and maintaining an alkaline PH is important for bodily health. If you are not completely satisfied with this product, the company will refund your money.

Index